# Collaborative Practice in Obstetrics and Gynecology

*Guest Editors*

RICHARD WALDMAN, MD
HOLLY POWELL KENNEDY, PhD

OBSTETRICS AND GYNECOLOGY CLINICS OF NORTH AMERICA

www.obgyn.theclinics.com

*Consulting Editor*
WILLIAM F. RAYBURN, MD, MBA

September 2012 • Volume 39 • Number 3

SAUNDERS an imprint of ELSEVIER, Inc.

**W.B. SAUNDERS COMPANY**
*A Division of Elsevier Inc.*

Elsevier, Inc. • 1600 John F. Kennedy Blvd. • Suite 1800 • Philadelphia, PA 19103-2899

http://www.theclinics.com

**OBSTETRICS AND GYNECOLOGY CLINICS OF NORTH AMERICA Volume 39, Number 3**
**September 2012 ISSN 0889-8545, ISBN-13: 978-1-4557-4900-3**

Editor: Stephanie Donley



*Obstetrics and Gynecology Clinics* (ISSN 0889-8545) is published quarterly by Elsevier Inc., 360 Park Avenue South, New York, NY 10010-1710. Months of issue are March, June, September, and December. Periodicals postage paid at New York, NY, and additional mailing offices. Subscription price per year is $275.00 (US individuals), $474.00 (US institutions), $137.00 (US students), $331.00 (Canadian individuals), $598.00 (Canadian institutions), $201.00 (Canadian students), $402.00 (foreign individuals), $598.00 (foreign institutions), and $201.00 (foreign students). To receive student/resident rate, orders must be accompanied by name of affiliated institution, date of term, and the signature of program/residency coordinator on institution letterhead. Orders will be billed at individual rate until proof of status is received. Foreign air speed delivery is included in all *Clinics* subscription prices. All prices are subject to change without notice. POSTMASTER: Send address changes to *Obstetrics and Gynecology Clinics*, Elsevier Health Sciences Division, Subscription Customer Service, 3251 Riverport Lane, Maryland Heights, MO 63043. **Customer Service: Telephone: 1-800-654-2452 (U.S. and Canada); 314-447-8871 (outside U.S. and Canada). Fax: 314-447-8029. E-mail: journalscustomerservice-usa@elsevier.com (for print support); journalsonlinesupport-usa@elsevier.com (for online support).**

*Reprints.* For copies of 100 or more of articles in this publication, please contact the Commercial Reprints Department, Elsevier Inc., 360 Park Avenue South, New York, New York 10010-1710. Tel.: 212-633-3818; Fax: 212-462-1935; E-mail: reprints@elsevier.com.

*Obstetrics and Gynecology Clinics of North America* is also published in Spanish by McGraw-Hill Interamericana Editores S.A., P.O. Box 5-237, 06500, Mexico; in Portuguese by Reichmann and Affonso Editores, Rio de Janeiro, Brazil; and in Greek by Paschalidis Medical Publications, Athens, Greece.

*Obstetrics and Gynecology Clinics of North America is covered in MEDLINE/PubMed (Index Medicus), Excerpta Medica, Current Concepts/Clinical Medicine, Science Citation Index, BIOSIS, CINAHL, and ISI/BIOMED.*

Printed and bound by CPI Group (UK) Ltd, Croydon, CR0 4YY

Transferred to Digital Print 2012

**GOAL STATEMENT**

The goal of *Obstetrics and Gynecology Clinics of North America* is to keep practicing physicians up to date with current clinical practice in OB/GYN by providing timely articles reviewing the state of the art in patient care.

**ACCREDITATION**

The *Obstetrics and Gynecology Clinics of North America* is planned and implemented in accordance with the Essential Areas and Policies of the Accreditation Council for Continuing Medical Education (ACCME) through the joint sponsorship of the University of Virginia School of Medicine and Elsevier. The University of Virginia School of Medicine is accredited by the ACCME to provide continuing medical education for physicians.

The University of Virginia School of Medicine designates this enduring material activity for a maximum of 15 *AMA PRA Category 1 Credit(s)*™ for each issue, 60 credits per year. Physicians should only claim credit commensurate with the extent of their participation in the activity.

The American Medical Association has determined that physicians not licensed in the US who participate in this CME enduring material activity are eligible for a maximum of 15 *AMA PRA Category 1 Credit*(s)™ for each issue, 60 credits per year.

Credit can be earned by reading the text material, taking the CME examination online at http://www.theclinics.com/home/cme, and completing the evaluation. After taking the test, you will be required to review any and all incorrect answers. Following completion of the test and evaluation, your credit will be awarded and you may print your certificate.

**FACULTY DISCLOSURE/CONFLICT OF INTEREST**

The University of Virginia School of Medicine, as an ACCME accredited provider, endorses and strives to comply with the Accreditation Council for Continuing Medical Education (ACCME) Standards of Commercial Support, Commonwealth of Virginia statutes, University of Virginia policies and procedures, and associated federal and private regulations and guidelines on the need for disclosure and monitoring of proprietary and financial interests that may affect the scientific integrity and balance of content delivered in continuing medical education activities under our auspices.

The University of Virginia School of Medicine requires that all CME activities accredited through this institution be developed independently and be scientifically rigorous, balanced and objective in the presentation/discussion of its content, theories and practices.

All authors/editors participating in an accredited CME activity are expected to disclose to the readers relevant financial relationships with commercial entities occurring within the past 12 months (such as grants or research support, employee, consultant, stock holder, member of speakers bureau, etc.). The University of Virginia School of Medicine will employ appropriate mechanisms to resolve potential conflicts of interest to maintain the standards of fair and balanced education to the reader. Questions about specific strategies can be directed to the Office of Continuing Medical Education, University of Virginia School of Medicine, Charlottesville, Virginia.

The faculty and staff of the University of Virginia Office of Continuing Medical Education have no financial affiliations to disclose.

**The authors/editors listed below have identified no professional or financial affiliations for themselves or their spouse/partner:**

Lisa Allee, CNM; Diane J. Angelini, EdD, CNM; Melissa D. Avery, PhD, CNM; Mary Paul Backman, CNM; Emily R. Baker, MD; May Hsieh Blanchard, MD; Emily Brandl-Salutz, MPH, MN, RN; Miriam N. Cordell, MSN, CNM; Donald R. Coustan, MD; Rebecca Cypher, MSN, PNNP; Stephanie Donley, (Acquisitions Editor); Sarah Egan, CNM, MS; Eve Espey, MD, MPH; Barbara Fildes, MS, CNM; Christina Flores, MD; Lisa Foglia, MD; Tina C. Foster, MD, MPH, MS; William Haffner, MD; Linda Heffner, MD, PhD; Jean Howe, MD, MPH; William Irvin, MD (Test Author); Holly Powell Kennedy, PhD, CNM (Guest Editor); Tekoa L. King, CNM, MPH; Abbe Kirsch, CNM, MS; Jan M. Kriebs, CNM, MSN; Russell K. Laros Jr, MD; Ruth Mankoff, CNM, MS; Nicole Marshall, CNM, NP, MS; Therese McMahan, CNM, MSN; Owen Montgomery, MD; Julie Mottl-Santiago, CNM, MPH; Michelle Munroe, CNM; Peter E. Nielsen, MD; Barbara O'Brien, MD; Joseph A. (Tony) Ogburn, MD; Julian T. Parer, MD, PhD; Christine Chang Pecci, MD; Roxanne I. Piecek, CNM; Marilyn Pierce-Bulger, CNM; William F. Rayburn, MD, MBA (Consulting Editor); Melissa Resnick, CNM, MS; Denise C. Smith, CNM; Richard Waldman, MD (Guest Editor); and Alan Waxman, MD, MPH.

**The authors/editors listed below identified the following professional or financial affiliations for themselves or their spouse/partner:**

**Dominic J. Cammarano III, DO** is employed by, and owns stock in, the Reading OB/GYN and Women's Birth Center.
**Larry Culpepper, MD, MPH** is on the Advisory Board for AstraZeneca, Forest Labs, Merck, Pfizer, Inc., and Takeda; and is on the Speakers' Bureau for Merck.
**Robin L. Grant, CNM, MSN** is employed by the Reading OB/GYN and Women's Birth Center.
**Susan Kendig, JD, MSN, WHNP-BC**'s spouse is employed by Latham Phillips Ophthalmic, and owns a family business, I Care Consulting.
**Aviva Lee-Parritz, MD**'s husband is employed by Sanofi.
**Janet Singer, MSN, CNM** owns stock in Sequenom, the Winslow Fund, and the Miller Howard Fund.
**Jennifer R. Stevens, CNM, MS** is employed by the Reading OB/GYN and Women's Birth Center and is on the Advisory Board for the American Association of Birth Centers.
**Tammy L. Witmer, CNM, MSN** is employed by the Reading OB/GYN and Women's Birth Center.

***Disclosure of Discussion of non-FDA approved uses for pharmaceutical products and/or medical devices:***

The University of Virginia School of Medicine, as an ACCME provider, requires that all faculty presenters identify and disclose any off-label uses for pharmaceutical and medical device products. The University of Virginia School of Medicine recommends that each physician fully review all the available data on new products or procedures prior to clinical use.

**TO ENROLL**

To enroll in the Obstetrics and Gynecology Clinics of North America Continuing Medical Education program, call customer service at 1-800-654-2452 or visit us online at www.theclinics.com/home/cme. The CME program is available to subscribers for an additional fee of $180.00.

# Contributors


## CONSULTING EDITOR

**WILLIAM F. RAYBURN, MD, MBA**
Randolph Seligman Professor and Chair, Department of Obstetrics and Gynecology; Chief of Staff, University Hospital, University of New Mexico Health Science Center, Albuquerque, New Mexico

## GUEST EDITORS

**RICHARD WALDMAN, MD, FACOG**
Past President, American College of Obstetricians and Gynecologists; Department of OB-GYN, SUNY Health Science Center, Syracuse, New York

**HOLLY POWELL KENNEDY, PhD, CNM, FACNM, FAAN**
President, American College of Nurse-Midwives, Silverspring, Maryland; Helen Varney Professor of Midwifery, Yale University School of Nursing, New Haven, Connecticut

## AUTHORS

**LISA ALLEE, CNM**
Northern Navajo Medical Center, Shiprock, New Mexico

**DIANE J. ANGELINI, EdD, CNM, FACNM, FAAN**
Clinical Professor, Department of Obstetrics and Gynecology; Director, Nurse Midwifery Section, Women & Infants Hospital of Rhode Island, Alpert Medical School of Brown University, Providence, Rhode Island

**MELISSA D. AVERY, PhD, CNM, FACNM, FAAN**
Professor, School of Nursing, University of Minnesota, Minneapolis, Minnesota

**MARY PAUL BACKMAN, CNM**
Staff Certified Nurse-Midwife, Madigan Army Medical Center, Tacoma, Washington

**EMILY R. BAKER, MD**
Director, Division of Maternal-Fetal Medicine, Department of Obstetrics and Gynecology, Dartmouth-Hitchcock Medical Center; Professor, Obstetrics and Gynecology, and Radiology, Dartmouth Medical School, Lebanon, New Hampshire

**MAY HSIEH BLANCHARD, MD, FACOG**
Associate Professor, Department of Obstetrics, Gynecology and Reproductive Sciences; Chief, Division of General Obstetrics and Gynecology, University of Maryland School of Medicine, Baltimore, Maryland

**EMILY BRANDL-SALUTZ, MPH, MN, RN**
School of Nursing, University of Minnesota, Minneapolis, Minnesota

**DOMINIC J. CAMMARANO III, DO, FACOG**
Medical Director and Owner, Reading OB/GYN and Women's Birth Center; Chief, Section of Gynecology, Reading Hospital and Medical Center, Reading, Pennsylvania

**MIRIAM N. CORDELL, MS, CNM**
Director, Division of Nurse Midwives and Practitioners, Department of Obstetrics and Gynecology, Dartmouth-Hitchcock Medical Center; Clinical Instructor, Obstetrics and Gynecology, Dartmouth Medical School, Lebanon, New Hampshire

**DONALD R. COUSTAN, MD**
Professor, Department of Obstetrics and Gynecology, Women & Infants Hospital of Rhode Island, Alpert Medical School of Brown University, Providence, Rhode Island

**LARRY CULPEPPER, MD, MPH**
Professor of Family Medicine, Boston University School of Medicine, Boston, Massachusetts

**REBECCA CYPHER, MSN, PNNP**
Perinatal Nurse Specialist, Madigan Army Medical Center, Tacoma, Washington

**SARAH EGAN, CNM, MS**
Midwife, Department of OB/GYN, Good Samaritan Hospital, Los Angeles, California; Planned Parenthood Pasadena/San Gabriel Valley, Pasadena, California

**EVE ESPEY, MD, MPH**
Professor and Chief of Family Planning, Department of Obstetrics and Gynecology, University of New Mexico, Albuquerque, New Mexico

**BARBARA FILDES, MS, CNM, FACNM**
Manager, Regional Obstetrics Improvement, New England Alliance for Health at Dartmouth Hitchcock Medical Center; Assistant Professor, Obstetrics and Gynecology, Dartmouth Medical School, Lebanon, New Hampshire

**CHRISTINA FLORES, MD**
Attending Physician/Medical Student Site Director, Department of OB/GYN, Bronx Lebanon Hospital Center, Bronx, New York

**LTC LISA FOGLIA, MD, FACOG**
MC, USA, Program Director, OB/GYN Residency Program, Madigan Army Medical Center, Tacoma, Washington

**TINA C. FOSTER, MD, MPH, MS**
Acting Director, Division of General Obstetrics and Gynecology, Dartmouth-Hitchcock Medical Center; Associate Professor, Obstetrics and Gynecology, and Community and Family Medicine, Dartmouth Medical School, Lebanon, New Hampshire

**ROBIN L. GRANT, CNM, MSN**
Clinical Director, Reading Birth and Women's Center; Clinical Director, Reading OB/GYN and Women's Birth Center, Reading, Pennsylvania; American College of Nurse Midwives, Silver Spring, Maryland; Commission for Accreditation of Birth Centers, Miami, Florida

**WILLIAM H.J. HAFFNER, MD**
Professor, Uniformed Services University of the Health Sciences, Bethesda, Maryland

**LINDA HEFFNER, MD, PhD**
Professor of Obstetrics and Gynecology, Boston University School of Medicine, Boston, Massachusetts

**JEAN HOWE, MD, MPH**
Northern Navajo Medical Center, Shiprock, New Mexico

**SUSAN KENDIG, JD, MSN, WHNP-BC, FAANP**
Associate Teaching Professor, Women's Health Nurse Practitioner, Emphasis Area Coordinator, University of Missouri College of Nursing, St Louis, Missouri

**HOLLY POWELL KENNEDY, PhD, CNM, FACNM, FAAN**
President, American College of Nurse-Midwives, Silverspring, Maryland; Helen Varney Professor of Midwifery, Yale University School of Nursing, New Haven, Connecticut

**TEKOA L. KING, CNM, MPH, FACNM**
Deputy Editor, Journal of Midwifery & Women's Health, Oakland, California

**ABBE KIRSCH, CNM, MS**
Assistant Director of Midwifery Services, Department of OB/GYN, Bronx Lebanon Hospital Center, Bronx, New York

**JAN M. KRIEBS, CNM, MSN, FACNM**
Assistant Professor, Department of Obstetrics, Gynecology and Reproductive Sciences; Director, Division of Midwifery, University of Maryland School of Medicine, Baltimore, Maryland

**RUSSELL K. LAROS Jr, MD, FACOG**
Professor, Department of Obstetrics, Gynecology and Reproductive Health, University of California, San Francisco, San Francisco, California

**AVIVA LEE-PARRITZ, MD**
Associate Professor of Obstetrics and Gynecology, Boston University School of Medicine; Vice Chair, Residency Program; Director, Department of Obstetrics and Gynecology, Boston Medical Center, Boston, Massachusetts

**RUTH MANKOFF, CNM, MS**
Director of Midwifery Services, Department of OB/GYN, Bronx Lebanon Hospital Center, Bronx, New York

**NICOLE MARSHALL, CNM, NP, MS**
Midwife, Department of OB/GYN, Elmhurst Hospital, Queens, New York; Clinical Research Nurse- Practitioner, Department of Medicine, Albert Einstein College of Medicine, Bronx, New York; Nurse Practitioner, Ottenheimer Healthcare, Manhattan, New York

**THERESE McMAHAN, CNM, MSN**
Staff Midwife, Cambridge Health Alliance, Cambridge, Massachusettes

**OWEN MONTGOMERY, MD, FACOG**
Chair, Department of Obstetrics and Gynecology, Drexel University, Philadelphia, Pennsylvania

**JULIE MOTTL-SANTIAGO, CNM, MPH**
Assistant Professor of Obstetrics and Gynecology, Boston University School of Medicine; Director of Midwifery Services, Department of Obstetrics and Gynecology, Boston Medical Center, Boston, Massachusetts

**LTC MICHELLE MUNROE, CNM**
AN, USA, Deputy Commander for Nursing, Kenner Army Health Clinic, Fort Lee, Virginia

**COL PETER E. NIELSEN, MD, FACOG**
MC, USA, Director, Clinical Operations, OB/GYN Consultant to The Surgeon General, Western Regional Medical Command, Washington

**BARBARA O'BRIEN, MD**
Assistant Professor, Department of Obstetrics and Gynecology, Women & Infants Hospital, Alpert Medical School of Brown University, Providence, Rhode Island

**JOSEPH A. (TONY) OGBURN, MD**
Professor and Chief of General Obstetrics and Gynecology, Department of Obstetrics and Gynecology, University of New Mexico, Albuquerque, New Mexico

**JULIAN T. PARER, MD, PhD, FACOG**
Professor, Department of Obstetrics, Gynecology and Reproductive Health, University of California, San Francisco, San Francisco, California

**CHRISTINE CHANG PECCI, MD**
Assistant Professor of Family Medicine, Boston University School of Medicine; Director of Maternal Child Health, Department of Family Medicine, Boston Medical Center, Boston, Massachusetts

**ROXANNE I. PIECEK, CNM**
Assistant Chief, Nurse-Midwifery Service, Madigan Army Medical Center, Tacoma, Washington

**MARILYN PIERCE-BULGER, CNM, FNP, MN**
Southcentral Foundation, Anchorage, Alaska

**MELISSA RESNICK, CNM, MS**
Midwife, Department of OB/GYN, Bronx Lebanon Hospital Center, Bronx, New York

**JANET SINGER, MSN, CNM**
Senior Clinical Teaching Associate, Department of Obstetrics and Gynecology, Women & Infants Hospital of Rhode Island, Alpert Medical School of Brown University, Providence, Rhode Island

**DENISE C. SMITH, CNM**
Certified Nurse-Midwife, PhD Student, College of Nursing, University of Colorado, Aurora, Colorado

**JENNIFER R. STEVENS, CNM, MS**
Administrative Director, Reading Birth and Women's Center; Vice President, American Association of Birth Centers; Administrative Director, Reading OB/GYN and Women's Birth Center, Reading, Pennsylvania; American College of Nurse Midwives, Silver Spring, Maryland; Commission for Accreditation of Birth Centers, Miami, Florida

**RICHARD WALDMAN, MD, FACOG**
Past President, American College of Obstetricians and Gynecologists; Department of OB-GYN, SUNY Health Science Center, Syracuse, New York

**ALAN WAXMAN, MD, MPH**
Professor, Department of Obstetrics and Gynecology, University of New Mexico, Albuquerque, New Mexico

**TAMMY L. WITMER, CNM, MSN**
Certified Nurse Midwife, Reading Birth and Women's Center; Reading OB/GYN and Women's Birth Center, Reading, Pennsylvania; American College of Nurse Midwives, Silver Spring, Maryland; Commission for Accreditation of Birth Centers, Miami, Florida

# Contents

**Foreword: Effective Collaboration** xvii

William F. Rayburn

**Preface: The Long and Winding Road to Effective Collaboration** xix

Richard Waldman and Holly Powell Kennedy

**The Birth of a Collaborative Model: Obstetricians, Midwives, and Family Physicians** 323

Christine Chang Pecci, Julie Mottl-Santiago, Larry Culpepper, Linda Heffner, Therese McMahan, and Aviva Lee-Parritz

In the United States, the challenges of maternity care include provider workforce, cost containment, and equal access to quality care. This article describes a collaborative model of care involving midwives, family physicians, and obstetricians at the Boston Medical Center, which serves a low-income multicultural population. Leadership investment in a collaborative model of care from the Department of Obstetrics and Gynecology, Section of Midwifery, and the Department of Family Medicine created a culture of safety and commitment to patient-centered care. Essential elements of the authors' successful model include a commitment to excellence in patient care, communication, and interdisciplinary education.

**Midwifery and Obstetrics: Twenty Years of Collaborative Academic Practice** 335

Diane J. Angelini, Barbara O'Brien, Janet Singer, and Donald R. Coustan

This review describes a collaborative educational practice model partnering midwifery and obstetrics within a department of obstetrics and gynecology. For more than 20 years, the authors' model has demonstrated sustainability and influence on medical education. The focus is on resident education in obstetrics, using midwifery faculty as teachers in the obstetric and obstetric triage settings. This noncompetitive and integrated educational practice model has achieved sustainability and success using midwives in a collaborative approach to medical education. The continuing collaboration and innovation within medical and resident education are important elements for the future of collaborative practice.

**Description of a Successful Collaborative Birth Center Practice Among Midwives and an Obstetrician** 347

Jennifer R. Stevens, Tammy L. Witmer, Robin L. Grant, and Dominic J. Cammarano III

Collaboration among professional groups is essential for safe and efficient health care. Midwifery care is optimized when allowed to function independently within an integrated health care system of support to address complications should they arise. A formal process for collaboration facilitates a smooth, expedient flow of information and decision making in a time of need, maximizing safety and efficiency. This article describes a successful collaborative model among four midwives and one obstetrician that addresses the impending maternity health care provider shortage, the needs of vulnerable populations, and cost-efficiency through appropriate use of technology and choice of health care provider.

**Midwives and Obstetrician-Gynecologists Collaborating for Native American Women's Health** **359**

Joseph A. (Tony) Ogburn, Eve Espey, Marilyn Pierce-Bulger, Alan Waxman, Lisa Allee, William Haffner, and Jean Howe

Certified Nurse-Midwives (CNMs) and Obstetrician-Gynecologists (OBGs) have a long history of successful collaborative practice serving Native American women from the 1960s. CNMs provide holistic, patient-centered care focusing on normal pregnancy and childbirth. OBGs support CNMs with consultation services focusing on complications during pregnancy and specialty gynecology care. Collaborative care in Indian Health Service and Tribal sites optimizes maternity care in a supportive environment, achieving excellent outcomes including low rates of cesarean deliveries and high rates of successful vaginal birth after cesarean.

**A Successful Model of Collaborative Practice in a University-Based Maternity Care Setting** **367**

May Hsieh Blanchard and Jan M. Kriebs

When building an integrated practice, the ability of each team member to work comfortably with other professionals is key. Midwives need to understand departmental expectations for participation in resident/student education, be willing to provide midwifery care in a high-acuity setting with limited opportunities for low-intervention care, and understand expectations for clinical leadership. Physicians need to build on the group expectation of mutual respect and best use of each group member. Confusion about midwifery and physician roles in maternity care still exists.

**Working Toward a Common Goal: A Collaborative Obstetrics and Gynecology Practice** **373**

Nicole Marshall, Sarah Egan, Christina Flores, Abbe Kirsch, Ruth Mankoff, and Melissa Resnick

Health care reform in the United States will continue to necessitate creativity in the organization and staffing of health care models. The Department of Obstetrics and Gynecology at Bronx-Lebanon Hospital Center has expanded its staff by placing midwives as primary providers for most routine care and much of the specialty care offered within the department. Midwives and attending physicians work collaboratively in outpatient specialty clinics. Inpatient care is provided by a team of midwives, residents, and attending physicians. This model of care is easily replicated, and has resulted in improvements in clinical practice and increased patient and personnel satisfaction.

**Collaborative Maternity Care: Three Decades of Success at Dartmouth-Hitchcock Medical Center** **383**

Miriam N. Cordell, Tina C. Foster, Emily R. Baker, and Barbara Fildes

This article describes the development of our collaborative practice, discusses the barriers and challenges presented by the current health care environment, and identifies factors that would encourage the initiation and strengthening of a successful collaborative model in similar settings. Successful collaborative practice is more than just a practice model, or a set of items that, once checked off, will guarantee success. It is a process that is inextricably linked to the focus and dedication of all our clinicians to provide the best care possible for women.

**Collaborative Practice Model: Madigan Army Medical Center** **399**

Peter E. Nielsen, Michelle Munroe, Lisa Foglia, Roxanne I. Piecek, Mary Paul Backman, Rebecca Cypher, and Denise C. Smith

In 2007, Madigan Army Medical Center implemented a new maternity care delivery model, integrating obstetricians and certified nurse-midwives (CNMs) in a collaborative practice. The change was driven by multiple factors, including patient preference, changes in the resident workweek, and low provider satisfaction. This article describes the elements of successful collaboration, including the structure, effective teamwork principles, role of the CNM in resident education, and preliminary data on mode of delivery, the number of CNM-supervised resident births, and procedures, such as episiotomy and epidural use.

**Interprofessional Collaborative Practice in Obstetrics and Midwifery** **411**

Tekoa L. King, Russell K. Laros Jr, and Julian T. Parer

As the health care system transforms to accommodate an increased need for primary care services and more patients, new models of health care delivery are needed that can provide quality health care services efficiently. An integrated collaborative practice of certified nurse-midwives, obstetrician-gynecologists, and perinatologists is best suited to meet the rapidly changing needs of the maternity health care delivery system. This article reviews the literature on interprofessional collaborative practice and describes the structure, function, and essential elements of successful collaboration in health care.

**Essential Components of Successful Collaborative Maternity Care Models: The ACOG-ACNM Project** **423**

Melissa D. Avery, Owen Montgomery, and Emily Brandl-Salutz

The American College of Obstetricians and Gynecologists (ACOG) and the American College of Nurse-Midwives (ACNM) asked ACNM member midwives and ACOG Fellows with successful and sustainable collaborative practices between obstetricians and midwives to describe their care models in jointly written articles. This review analyzes 12 of the 60 articles submitted. Five main themes were identified: impetus for new collaboration, basic foundations of collaborative care, commitment to successful partnership, care integration, and health professions education in an interprofessional practice environment. The analysis provides evidence of the extent to which committed clinicians are working together to provide excellent, women-centered maternity care.

**Collaboration in Maternity Care: Possibilities and Challenges** **435**

Richard Waldman, Holly Powell Kennedy, and Susan Kendig

The United States is about to face a maternity workforce crisis in the next decade because the number of medical students choosing obstetrics and gynecology is stagnant, the number of patients requiring care is increasing and many in the current workforce of obstetricians/gynecologists and midwives are ready to retire. There are not enough maternity providers to meet the future needs of women. Creative strategies must be explored to address these concerns. Collaborative practice among different types of maternity providers requires commitment, interpersonal skills, and teamwork. This article explores these issues and provides practical tips and a case study of the process in action between the American College of Obstetricians and Gynecologists and the American College of Nurse-Midwives.

**Index** **445**

# OBSTETRICS AND GYNECOLOGY CLINICS

## FORTHCOMING ISSUES

***December 2012***
**Medical and Surgical Management of Common Fertility Issues**
G. Wright Bates Jr, MD, *Guest Editor*

***March 2013***
**Obstetric Emergencies**
James Alexander, MD, Carolyn Y. Muller, MD and Michael P. Traynor, MD, MPH, *Guest Editors*

***June 2013***
**Colposcopy and Cervical Cancer Screening**
Alan Waxman, MD and Maria Lina Diaz, MD, *Guest Editors*

## RECENT ISSUES

***June 2012***
**Update of Gynecologic Oncology**
Carolyn Y. Muller, MD

***March 2012***
**Management of Preterm Birth: Best Practices in Prediction, Prevention, and Treatment**
Alice Reeves Goepfert, MD, *Guest Editor*

***December 2011***
**Advances in Laparoscopy and Minimally Invasive Surgery**
Michael P. Traynor, MD, MPH

# Foreword
# Effective Collaboration

This issue of *Obstetrics and Gynecology Clinics of North America,* co-edited by Dr Holly Kennedy and Dr Richard Waldman, deals with a nontraditional yet very important subject pertaining to effective collaboration between obstetricians and certified nurse midwives. In light of health care reform and presumed shortages of physicians, interprofessional collaboration is to be championed as a critical strategy for improving health care outcomes. The medical literature documents the benefits of coordinated team care to improve outcomes in acute care settings and for delivery of preventive services. This evidence has increased awareness that such collaboration will be an important part in creating a safer and more effective health care system.

Despite this emerging evidence, collaborative efforts have not been adopted universally across health professions unless resources require it. Recognizing the need and potential for more effective collaboration, this issue examines how a variety of settings—academic health care centers, community settings, and private practices—are implementing these models. Graduate and continuing education play essential roles. Highlighted in this issue are experiences of several participating institutions to compare and contrast their provision of patient-centered care.

As mentioned by the guest editors, building a nonhierarchical relation between ob-gyns and nurse midwives can liberate any tensions between professionals and unleash the power to be an effective team. Collaboration that works well is no accident, since the act is a repetitive process. We need to be proactive in outlining a future that guarantees women and their families to have qualified maternity providers at their births and access to excellent preventive health care.

Interprofessional education and interactions should begin early. Portions of this issue provide an introduction to integrative educational models in graduate training as opportunities to build relationships, so that teamwork is shaped at the earliest stage of a student's learning. The authors describe processes and lessons learned at their respective institutions that are critical in the process of adopting collaboration programs. Building blocks at each institution include the planning processes, competencies to instill, and assessment strategies. We need more research to market models of collaborative practice that really work and are cost effective.

I would encourage obstetricians and midwives to join together at local and global levels to share in policy development, continuing education, research, and, most of all, preparation of the future maternity care workforce. Transforming the women's health care workforce will entail more teamwork and the inclusion of other nonphysician clinicians such as advanced nurse practitioners and physician assistants who can perform clinical tasks and assist on procedures. It is noteworthy that their emergence as a strong presence in the workforce grew out of the market reconfiguration in the 1980s produced by managed health care.

Obstet Gynecol Clin N Am 39 (2012) xvii–xviii
http://dx.doi.org/10.1016/j.ogc.2012.08.001
0889-8545/12/$ – see front matter  

Information in this issue represents the experience and opinions of many thoughtful leaders in maternity care. Their contributions are important, especially in addressing the patient's preconceived impressions and in providing certain articles that contain useful educational materials. While views expressed here are not absolute, guidelines described in this issue should serve as further evidence in addressing our patient-centered workforce needs.

William F. Rayburn, MD, MBA
Department of Obstetrics and Gynecology
University of New Mexico School of Medicine
MSC10 5580; 1 University of New Mexico
Albuquerque, NM 87131-0001, USA

E-mail address:
wrayburn@salud.unm.edu

# Preface

# The Long and Winding Road to Effective Collaboration

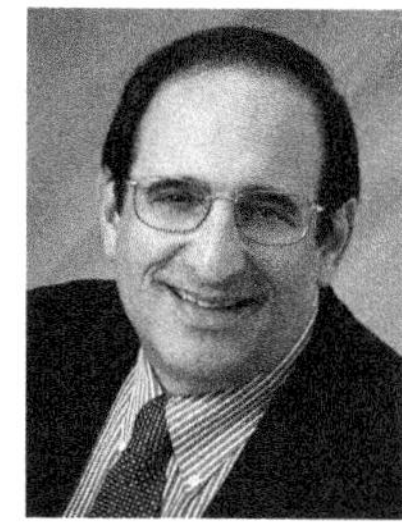

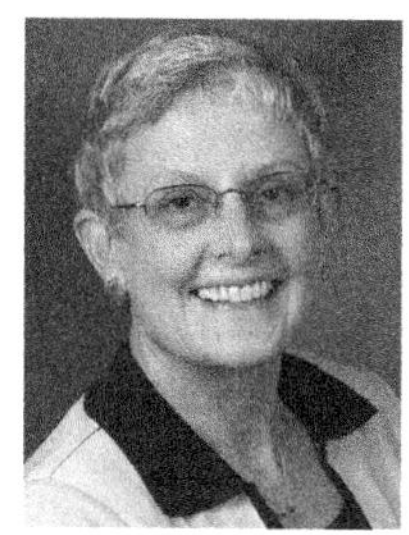

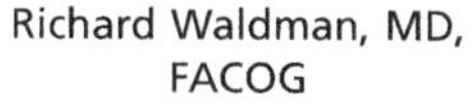
Richard Waldman, MD, FACOG

Holly Powell Kennedy, PhD, CNM, FACNM, FAAN

*Guest Editors*

Why have we devoted an entire issue to the topic of collaboration among obstetricians and midwives? Quite simply, the supply of maternity providers is diminishing, which will compromise women's access to quality health care. A global view of maternity care in the United States reveals some serious design flaws. The physician work force is poorly distributed, is in short supply, and is predicted to erode further. Many births occur in hospitals with less than 1000 births per year and are struggling to provide an adequate supply of qualified providers. More than 9.5 million Americans live in counties that lack obstetricians—half of all counties in the United States. We are increasingly challenged to provide care in our inner cities and our rural communities. The pipeline that prepares obstetricians, certified nurse midwives (CNM), and certified midwives (CM) is frozen at 20th century levels. It is time to collaborate in the redesign of maternity care and to address the projected shortages of maternity providers together.

As we look to the future of maternity care, we must be strategic in education, practice, policy, and research. Although nurse practitioner and physician assistant ranks have dramatically increased, the number of CNM/CMs and obstetrical residents lags behind. There must be a concerted expeditious effort to increase our cohort of maternity providers while maintaining quality and controlling cost. It will require innovative and interdisciplinary creativity to work as equal partners, each contributing valued service to the maternity care team.

During the last two years, the American College of Obstetricians and Gynecologists (ACOG) and the American College of Nurse-Midwives (ACNM) have consciously improved our collaborative intelligence. We produced a new statement on joint practice relations,[1] had our presidents attend each others' executive board meetings, and shared a project to showcase collaborative models of care that work.

Obstet Gynecol Clin N Am 39 (2012) xix–xxii
http://dx.doi.org/10.1016/j.ogc.2012.07.001 

The latter project called for articles describing collaborative OB/GYN and CNM/CM practices—60 teams answered the challenge. Four of those articles were published in the *Green Journal* in late 2011.[2-5] This issue of *Obstetrics and Gynecology Clinics of North America* presents 11 articles chosen for merit and breadth. They describe a wide range of practices across the United States in community settings, academic centers, private practice, and locations devoted to the care of vulnerable women. Overwhelmingly, there is a sense of pride and camaraderie as the authors describe the interdisciplinary work, their challenges, and their successes. In the last article, Avery, Montgomery, and Brandle-Salutz provide a qualitative analysis of all articles submitted to synthesize common areas of collaboration.

As we were putting the issue together, a graduate student midwife in one of the settings described in this article shared the experience of her first day in working with the interdisciplinary team. She gave us permission to publish her journal entry in our editorial since it captured the essence of what should be happening during the educational process of a new generation of maternity providers and the value of teaching and learning at all levels.

> *Boston Medical Center (BMC) has lived up to its reputation of offering women (and students) an integrated midwifery-obstetrics-family medicine department. The midwives practice side-by-side as attending [providers] with the obstetricians and family medicine MDs, precepting residents in inpatient and outpatient settings, and serving as faculty at Boston University School of Medicine ... the midwives and obstetricians constantly consulted and rounded with each other about all of the patients on the floor with collegiality and respect.*
>
> *... the residents not only welcomed me with open arms but also immediately began carving out clinical opportunities for me, including me in their conversations about patients and even offering me birth opportunities. The first baby I caught at BMC was a woman who was a continuity patient of one of the residents. The resident, who had stayed three hours post-call for this woman's birth, allowed me to be the primary catcher... she precepted me as we were both precepted by my midwifery preceptor, the attending [provider] for the patient. Then, after watching a painstakingly slow hour of my novice suturing work, the same resident thanked me for giving her the opportunity to teach. It is the first time someone has ever said that to me during my training as a midwife and I love the significance such a statement gives to the importance of teaching (Erin George, RN, Yale School of Nursing Midwifery Student, January, 2012)*

Our efforts in designing this issue, and our work over the past two years, were initially focused on improving the relationship between ACOG and ACNM. Many of us believe the effort at building a nonhierarchical relationship actually liberated the tension that had existed between our organizations and unleashed the power of an effective team. Treating ourselves with respect at the organizational level created a harmonious collaborative spirit that allowed our two organizations dedicated to improving women's health care to accomplish so much more together. We spent less and less time in tense negotiations defending turf and much more time on working together on the future needs of women. We are now working together on many more projects addressing the health of women and their families in all settings.

Collaboration that works well is no accident since the act is a recursive process. We need to be proactive in outlining a future that guarantees that women and families have qualified maternity providers at their births and access to superb women's health care throughout their lives. Collaboration and professional communication need to take a more prominent role in our educational programs. Integrative educational models should be explored as opportunities to build relationships, so that teamwork is shaped at the earliest stage of a student's learning. Lack of understanding of disciplinary values, knowledge, skills, and scope of practice is a major hurdle to effective team function. Student applicants should also be evaluated on their ability to work on a team. Top candidates who are not team players will not integrate well into a collaborative system. The idea is not to attract a star but rather to attract someone who is a star, but who can work effectively with an interdisciplinary team.

We need research that dissects and markets models of collaborative practice that work. We also need to plan for the future of maternity care by ensuring access to qualified maternity providers, in addition to understanding which models are most cost effective. This requires more midwifery educational programs and the elimination of state laws and hospital policies that obstruct the practice of well-educated midwives. Finally, we would encourage the obstetricians and midwives to join together at local and global levels to share in policy development, continuing education, research, and most of all preparation of the future maternity care workforce. In doing so, we have an opportunity to create a just world for women in which they have access to a cadre of skilled maternity providers. Perhaps the words of Martin Luther King, Jr best summarize this process of collaboration: "True peace is not merely the absence of tension: it is the presence of justice."[6]

Richard Waldman, MD, FACOG
American College of Obstetricians and Gynecologists
770 James Street
Syracuse, NY 13203, USA

Holly Powell Kennedy, PhD, CNM, FACNM, FAAN
American College of Nurse-Midwives
8403 Colesville Road
Suite 1550
Silver Spring, MD 20910-6374, USA

E-mail addresses:
rwacog@aol.com (R. Waldman)
holly.kennedy@yale.edu (H.P. Kennedy)

## REFERENCES

1. ACNM & ACOG, 2011, Joint Satement of Practice Relations Between Obstetrician-Gynecologists and Certified Nurse-midwives/Certified midwives. Silver Spring (MD): American College of Nurse-Midwives. Available at: http://www.midwife.org/ACNM/files/ACNMLibraryData/UPLOADFILENAME/000000000224/ACNM.ACOG%20Joint%20Statement%203.30.11.pdf. Accessed August 18, 2012.
2. Darlington A, McBroom K, Warwick S. A northwest collaborative practice model. Obstetrics & Gynecology 2011;118(3):673–7.
3. DeJoy S, Burkman RT, Graves BW, et al. Making it work: successful collaborative practice. Obstetrics & Gynecology 2011;118(3):683–6.
4. Hutchison MS, Ennis L, Shaw-Battista J, et al. Great minds don't think alike: collaborative maternity care at San Francisco General Hospital. Obstetrics & Gynecology 2011;118(3):678–82.
5. Shaw-Battista J, Fineberg A, Boehler B, et al. Obstetrician and nurse-midwife collaboration: successful public health and private practice partnership. Obstetrics & Gynecology 2011;118(3):663–72.

6. King ML. Letter from Birmingham City Jail, Birmingham, AL. April 16 1963. Available at: http://www.thekingcenter.org/archive/list?keys=True+peace+is+not+merely+the+absence+of+tension%3A+it+is+the+presence+of+justice&field_datetime_value%5Bvalue%5D%5Byear%5D=1963&field_datetime_value%5Bvalue%5D%5Bmonth%5D=4&field_datetime_value%5Bvalue%5D%5Bday%5D=16&field_datetime_value_1%5Bvalue%5D%5Byear%5D=&field_datetime_value_1%5Bvalue%5D%5Bmonth%5D=&field_datetime_value_1%5Bvalue%5D%5Bday%5D=&field_term_genre_tid=All&field_creationplace_value=&field_term_organization_tid=&field_term_person_tid=&field_publication_value=&field_term_topic_tid=&field_term_web_theme_tid=&=Submit. Accessed February 6, 2012.

# The Birth of a Collaborative Model

## Obstetricians, Midwives, and Family Physicians

Christine Chang Pecci, MD[a,*], Julie Mottl-Santiago, CNM, MPH[a], Larry Culpepper, MD, MPH[a], Linda Heffner, MD, PhD[a], Therese McMahan, CNM, MSN[b], Aviva Lee-Parritz, MD[a]

**KEYWORDS**

• Collaborative model • Midwives • Obstetricians • Family physicians

**KEY POINT**

- The design and implementation of a collaborative model of intrapartum care that involves obstetricians, midwives, and family physicians are described.

Those organizing maternity care in the United States face major challenges, including the impending shortage of obstetricians and consequent limitations in access to quality perinatal care for some populations.[1–3] Family physicians and certified nurse-midwives provide labor and delivery services in some communities and may offer solutions by addressing provider workforce, access to care, and cost issues in maternity care. These provider groups deliver safe care[4–6] while offering a diverse set of skills and expanded choices for women in childbirth.[7–15] Benefits of collaborative care include a more robust workforce with a better work-life balance, improved access to care and choice of providers, as well as appropriate care providers for individual patient needs.[16]

A unique collaboration among obstetricians, midwives, and family physicians at Boston Medical Center and its affiliated community health center network is described. Included is the evolution from 3 silos of individual professional practices characterized by interdisciplinary mistrust, inconsistent communication, and variable skill sets to a high-functioning, collaborative maternity care team with a clearly defined practice structure, sustainable systems that promote a culture of safety, and interdisciplinary education that integrates the skills and expertise of each profession.

The American College of Nurse-Midwives and the American Academy of Family Physicians each have joint statements with the American College of Obstetrics and

---

Presented in part at the Society of Teachers of Family Medicine Annual Spring Conference, Chicago, April 25–29, 2007.

[a] Boston Medical Center, Boston University School of Medicine, 1 Boston Medical Center Place, Boston, MA 02118, USA; [b] Cambridge Health Alliance, 1493 Cambridge Street, Cambridge, MA 02139, USA

* Corresponding author. Department of Family Medicine, Boston Medical Center, Boston University School of Medicine, 1 Boston Medical Center Place, Boston, MA 02118.

*E-mail address:* Christine.pecci@bmc.org

Obstet Gynecol Clin N Am 39 (2012) 323–334

http://dx.doi.org/10.1016/j.ogc.2012.05.001 **obgyn.theclinics.com**

0889-8545/12/$ – see front matter 

Gynecology emphasizing the importance of collaboration.[17,18] However, conflict, disruptive behavior, resentment, and lack of respect among intrapartum providers are not uncommon.[19–21] Successful models of collaborative maternity care must promote a work culture that builds trust and emphasizes interdisciplinary communication. Practitioner competence, accountability, risk-taking and assertiveness, willingness and ability to challenge assumptions, and critical self-reflection are necessary for diverse providers to work together collaboratively.[22–24] Robust systems for conflict resolution, opportunities for participation and building cohesion, effective communication, and mutual trust are necessary for a collaborative model. Interdisciplinary education is also an important element of successful working relationships.[25–27]

Effective collaboration and communication through teamwork can improve maternity care by preventing error.[28–35] In an effort to improve patient outcomes, some hospitals have implemented team training programs to improve interdisciplinary professional communication. Commitment to a culture of safety, interdisciplinary participation and flat hierarchy, effective leadership, and robust communication techniques are essential elements in the Agency for Research and Health care Quality's TeamSTEPPS training program.[35] These programs have succeeded in establishing authentic collaboration and cultures of safety.[32] Clarity regarding consultation and referral in collaborative care is also crucial.[36]

Boston Medical Center is a 508-bed tertiary care hospital affiliated with the Boston University School of Medicine that includes in its mission the provision of safety net services to the Boston region. The maternity unit includes 8 labor and delivery rooms, 5 triage beds, 7 high-risk antepartum beds, 2 operating rooms, and 2 postanesthesia recovery beds. In 2010, the maternity unit cared for approximately 2500 women giving birth and provided 2800 outpatient triage visits. Boston Medical Center serves an ethnically diverse population, including a maternal population that is 45% African American, Afro-Caribbean, Haitian, and African; 30% Latina; 15% White; and 10% other, including Asian and Middle Eastern. The majority (81%) of intrapartum patients are covered by government-sponsored health insurance. Boston Medical Center's mission to improve the health of vulnerable populations is reflected in its commitment to providing neighborhood-centered health services through a network of 16 urban community health centers. More than half (54%) of the intrapartum patients receive prenatal care at 1 of these centers. In addition, the hospital provides a robust interpreter services department and a multicultural doula program.

## BACKGROUND FOR THE INITIATION OF THE AUTHORS' COLLABORATIVE MODEL

Before the establishment of the collaborative model, we practiced in 3 silos of care. An obstetrician, a midwife, and a family physician each provided attending coverage for his or her own service. Similar to many academic settings, in-house obstetricians supervised deliveries by residents and covered emergencies as needed. Midwives, who are faculty members of the Department of Obstetrics and Gynecology, provided continuous 24-hour labor and delivery care for patients who received midwifery care antenatally. Intrapartum guidelines for consultation or transfer of care of midwifery patients with high-risk conditions or for operative delivery were clearly defined. However, mistrust and lack of respect between midwives and obstetricians created a culture that discouraged communication. Midwives worried that their patients would receive unnecessary interventional or operative care from the obstetricians whereas obstetricians worried that midwives would not consult in a timely manner. Evidence-based discussions about labor management between midwives and obstetricians often were not resolved to the satisfaction of either party. Residents and students gained minimal appreciation for midwifery care because interactions were limited to situations that required the assistance of a physician.

Family physicians were physically present on the unit only when an antenatal patient of a family physician was in active labor. Admissions to family medicine occurred less than once a day on an average, and their patients comprised only 10% of total deliveries. There was a wide variation of skills among the family physicians, between new residency graduates and fellowship-trained family physicians privileged to perform cesarean deliveries. Delivery volume also varied greatly among family physicians, with some attending fewer than 5 deliveries a year. Guidelines for consultation between family physicians and obstetricians were not clearly defined, and the culture did not encourage early consultation. A lack of presence and consistency in the competence of family physicians led to disrespect, mistrust, and poor communication with obstetricians, midwives, residents, and nurses.

Each professional provided patient care independently with minimal interaction unless there was a need for consultation. There was no awareness or discussion on how specific patient care interventions might affect the workload or flow on the unit. There was no cross coverage, leading to delays in clinical care if one provider was occupied. Review of adverse outcomes consisted of assigning blame to a single provider rather than examining systems of care that contributed to the poor outcome.

Educational activities also were disjointed and at times, reflected disrespect between disciplines. A first-year and a senior obstetrics resident were assigned to labor and delivery, except for 3 months of the year when 2 first-year residents of family medicine replaced the first-year residents of obstetrics. Midwifery students worked with the midwives with little interaction with the resident or attending physicians, unless they were seeking a consultation from an attending obstetrician. Residents were responsible for admission, evaluation, writing orders, labor management, and delivery of all physician patients; however, they were not involved in the care of midwifery patients except those transferred to the on-call obstetrician.

An anticipated increase in prenatal registration of approximately 400 deliveries from 1 of our of affiliated health centers and a concern that this volume change would lead to adverse perinatal outcomes prompted the leadership of obstetrics and gynecology, including its midwives, and the family medicine department, to address changes that could improve perinatal outcomes, patient safety, patient satisfaction, and graduate medical education.

In the fall of 2005, a multidisciplinary working group of obstetricians, family physicians, midwives, nurses, and residents met weekly to define a new model of collaborative care for patients on labor and delivery. The mission was to provide safe, high-quality, patient-centered care at all times. The new Collaborative Model for Excellence on Labor and Delivery elaborates 10 principles to ensure patient safety, provide efficient and excellent patient care, as well as strengthen education of the residents (**Box 1**). In July 2006, the model was formally introduced to all providers and nurses, and a large poster with the guiding principles was displayed on the labor and delivery units. For the first year of the project, the working group met weekly to address challenges and ensure the successful continued implementation of the model.

## THE PRACTICE MODEL

Leaders in the Department of Obstetrics and Gynecology, its Section of Midwifery, and the Department of Family Medicine envisioned the creation of a consistent complement of providers on labor and delivery, each contributing distinct expertise

**Box 1**
**Collaborative Model Principles**

**Principles of a Collaborative Labor & Delivery Team of Excellence and Patient Safety at Boston Medical Center**

**Mission:** *To provide safe, high quality, patient centered care at all times through adherence to the following principles:*

*1. Team Focused*

Responsibility for care of women in triage, during labor and delivery, and during their postpartum stay rests with a team of professionals rather than a single provider.

*2. Clarity of Responsibility*

The identity of the supervising provider and the team responsible for each case will be clear to all L&D staff at all times.

*3. Citizenship*

Interactions between partners will be respectful and constructive. Excellence in patient care will be the focus of communication. All providers will perform patient care, order entry and chart documentation. Frequent physical presence on the L&D area will promote communication and collaboration among providers.

*4. Acceptable Case Load*

Safe patient care is possible only if there are well rested providers responsible for a reasonable number of women in labor. No provider will be directly responsible for more than 3 women needing active management at any one time. If a provider caseload exceeds this number then the FM and OB attendings and CNM will huddle to reallocate the case loads.

*5. Maximizing Continuity*

The first option for assignment of the care provider on L&D is the provider group with whom the woman has developed an established relationship during prenatal care. Information will flow smoothly from the prenatal to L&D and postpartum and nursery providers, and to the site and providers of post-hospital mother and infant care.

*6. Frequent Communication*

Frequent communication is needed for safe provision of care and is promoted by regular interdisciplinary board rounds, ad hoc interdisciplinary updates with changes in plans or transfer among providers due to a change in risk status or patient load, team members cross-covering for one another when needed.

*7. Good Documentation*

There will be clear and consistent documentation of all care delivered. Co-management or transfer of care from one team to another will be stated in the chart.

*8. High Efficiency*

Providers should maximize the use of their skill set by caring for women whose needs match their highest level of training. The provider with the highest level of training should be caring for those women who need the highest level of care. Providers with a higher level of training should NOT be caring for women who can be cared for by professionals whose training is especially suited for those patient characteristics and preferences.

*9. Evidence-Based Care*

Care provided will be based on the current evidence, standardized from one provider to another, and be informed by a rigorous continuous quality improvement process.

*10. Excellence in Education*

As a teaching hospital, all team members have responsibility for the education of residents, students and other trainees.

in patient care. Family physicians could bring to the team expertise in managing medical conditions; midwives, expertise in managing normal labor and birth; and obstetricians, expertise in high-risk conditions and surgical management. To accomplish this mission, the Department of Family Medicine initiated a 24-hour continuous attending presence on labor and delivery. The midwives and obstetricians continued to provide continuous coverage of labor and delivery.

In 2007, a new algorithm for the distribution of intrapartum patients was introduced. Specifically, some patients who had been cared for by an obstetrician antenatally were assigned to the family physician (**Fig. 1**). This new algorithm increased the volume of vaginal deliveries for the family physicians and allowed the obstetricians to focus on patients at high risk and operative deliveries. Because the midwifery group already carried a substantial antenatal patient panel, their delivery volume remained stable and robust.

In addition, our process for distribution of patients in labor and delivery is patient centered and considers the specific needs of each woman. The diversity in provider staff mirrors our multicultural patients who may benefit by having a provider with relevant cultural or linguistic competence. Women who desire to labor without pain medications or with less intervention may choose to be placed on the midwifery service regardless of their type of prenatal provider.

Our collaborative model emphasizes care of the patient by a team of maternity care providers rather than a single provider. Obstetricians, family physicians, midwives, and residents together review patient history, care plans, and fetal tracings on every patient at formal teaching rounds in the morning and evening and informally throughout the day. This emphasis on frequent communication encourages early collaboration and discussion regarding evidence-based plans of care for each patient. All members of the team are encouraged to express their opinions and concerns; respectful communication is expected. The skill sets of each provider group are also maximized in our model (**Fig. 2**). Midwives attend 44% of vaginal deliveries and provide labor management for 12% of operative deliveries. This translates to a 10% cesarean birth rate for the midwifery service. Obstetricians focus on operative deliveries. The mixture of vaginal and operative deliveries for family physicians reflects the ratio of clinical skills provided this provider group. Family physicians with operative privileges provide labor and delivery coverage 70% of the time, whereas family physicians who attend only vaginal deliveries provide coverage 30% of the time.

Our triage unit also functions collaboratively. During weekday hours, an additional nurse-midwife dedicated to the triage unit evaluates patients and consults with the obstetrician or family physician when needed. During the night and weekends, the

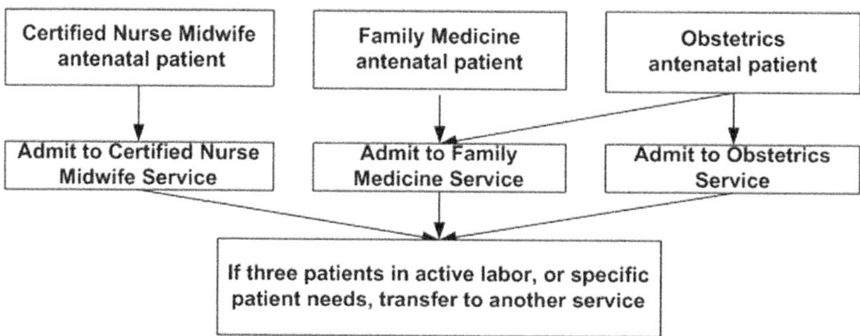


**Fig. 1.** Distribution of patients in labor and delivery.

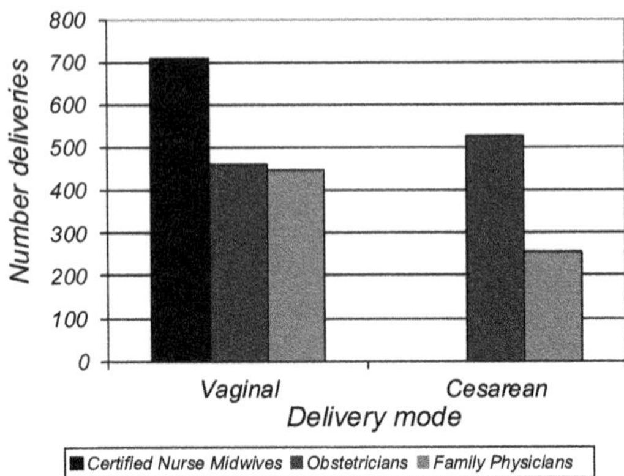


**Fig. 2.** Number and mode of deliveries by provider type (Jan 2010 to Dec 2010). Grid represents midwives, white dots on black bar represents obstetricians, black dots on white bar represents family physicians.

residents evaluate triage patients and then seek supervision from the midwife, family physician, or obstetrician, as appropriate.

## CHALLENGES AND SOLUTIONS

We faced challenges in establishing the principles of our collaborative model (see **Box 1**). Weekly meetings were crucial in stimulating collaborative discussions and proposals for changes to address issues. We describe some of our solutions here with acknowledgment that we continue to meet regularly to identify and respond to issues that arise.

Each provider group was challenged in a unique way during the implementation of our model. Leadership commitment was crucial for the success of our model. Leaders among all groups, including the chair and vice chair of both departments and the midwifery service director, championed this change with increased clinical time on labor and delivery. Each group provided guidance and accountability for their own faculty members.

Obstetricians were required to develop new skills on leadership that fostered participation and trust among all labor and delivery staff by reassessing the role of hierarchy in maternity care. Regular department workshops that focus on leadership development and communication skills have helped obstetrician faculty develop these skills.

The Department of Family Medicine required its physicians to achieve and maintain competence in intrapartum skills. This goal was accomplished by reducing the number of attendings participating in intrapartum care to only those with a strong interest in this area of practice and then engaging this group in an appraisal of skills. For 3 months, the department sponsored a weekly faculty seminar to review clinical topics and hands-on skills to refresh knowledge. Thereafter, monthly meetings of family physicians have addressed both administrative and clinical issues. The family medicine group now attends 30% of total deliveries, which is more than sufficient volume for maintenance of clinical skills.

Both obstetrician and family medicine attendings learned principles of citizenship, which requires all individuals to assist with patient-care tasks regardless of hierarchy. Attendings are expected to be visibly present and accessible, not off the floor or in call rooms, physically removed and disconnected from patient activities. Attendings are expected to participate in evaluating patients in triage, assisting with order entry, writing admission records or discharge summaries, and consenting patients for care because a delay in any of these tasks might affect the efficiency of care and patient safety. The departmental leadership addressed the behavior of individuals who did not engage in the expected citizenship or contribute to teamwork.

Stepping into a leadership and teaching role on the labor floor was a challenge for the midwives. Midwives had to adopt a more open and assertive communication style to promote evidence-based dialog with physician staff regarding patient care. Midwives were accustomed to interacting with the physicians and residents only when requesting a consultation, rather than participating in collaborative discussions around all intrapartum patients. Communication drills and modeling from the midwifery service director helped midwives build these skills. Regular group case reviews, discussion on new literature, and creation of a reading packet on normal birth for residents also improved the ability of the midwives to articulate the scientific evidence for their decisions.

Initially, both midwives and residents resisted midwifery involvement in resident education. Some midwives relished one-on-one patient care and were reluctant to include residents in all their births. Residents often had a busy load and would become preferentially less involved with midwifery patients. Persistent encouragement from the leadership and resident teaching workshops organized by both the obstetricians and the midwives has changed those dynamics. The midwifery service relished the opportunity to share its expertise in normal birth and nurtured future physician consultants.

## FINANCIAL CONSIDERATIONS

Safely staffing labor and delivery with midwives and family physicians is cost effective because of the differentials in professional liability premiums and salary. The addition of another in-house attending-level providers on labor and delivery required considerable planning and thoughtfulness. To emphasize teamwork and remove dysfunctional financial incentives among providers, the department chairs merged the billing for the care of all patients under a single entity, which reimburses each department for attending time on labor and delivery. Hospital leadership agreed to support this model financially. The total compensation (salary, fringe, malpractice, and continuing medical education) to add a continuous family medicine attending presence on labor and delivery is approximately $1.2 million, a considerable savings over adding a second obstetrician. This increased expense has been offset by a reduction in malpractice claims. Boston Medical Center is self-insured, therefore any savings in malpractice is directly beneficial to the institution. Our collaborative practice is one of several changes that have contributed to a steady and significant decrease in adverse perinatal outcomes and malpractice claims (**Fig. 3**).[37]

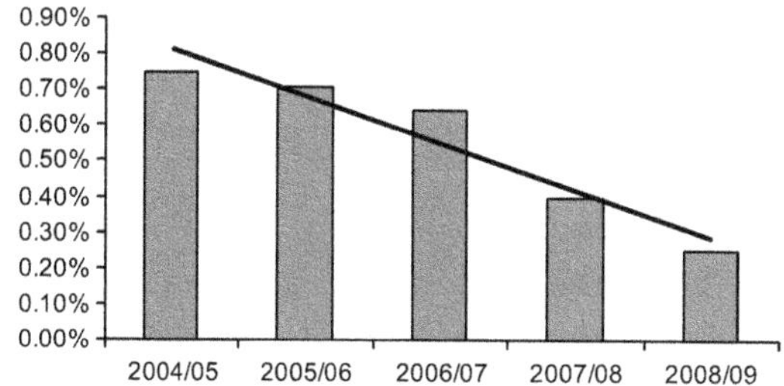


**Fig. 3.** Rate of reserved claims per policy year deliveries.

## BENEFITS OF THE INTERDISCIPLINARY TEAM MODEL

### *Culture of Safety*

One of the primary goals in the development of the collaborative model was to improve clinical outcomes by establishing a culture of safety. Breaking down our individual silos of care led to Team Training initiatives, and uniform competency requirements for providers. A multidisciplinary group of obstetricians, midwives, family physicians, anesthesiologists, and nurses participated in the Team Performance Plus team training course, which includes modules on communication and mutual respect. All physicians, midwives, nurses, and residents who are new at the authors' institution are required to attend this course. The obstetrics and family medicine departments agreed to the same minimum threshold of clinical activity by physicians and midwives for maintaining competence. They also collaboratively developed a standard to directly observe every faculty member joining the labor and delivery unit. In addition, on-line educational modules about fetal monitoring interpretation and emergency drills were established and members of all 3 services are mandated to participate and complete skill evaluations.

### *Patient-Focused Care*

Since the institution of our model, patient satisfaction has increased as measured by Press Ganey's Hospital Consumer Assessment of Health care Providers and Systems, a national public-reporting instrument (**Fig. 4**). In addition, the need to educate patients about our new labor and delivery model of care led to an interdisciplinary project to create a patient booklet that includes education about the prenatal, labor, birth, and postpartum periods. The midwives spearheaded the project with obstetricians, family physicians, nurses, and community doulas, all contributing to the content of this booklet. This booklet is given to all prenatal patients planning delivery at Boston Medical Center, regardless of type of the prenatal care provider.

### *Interdisciplinary Education*

Based on our new model, each laboring woman, including those cared for by midwives, has a first-year resident, or midwife student involved in her care. The addition of midwifery deliveries increased resident deliveries by 25%. Therefore the family medicine department modified its residency schedule to assign 1 family medicine first-year resident each month to labor and delivery year-round in addition to the already existing obstetrics and gynecology first-year resident. The first-year residents of family medicine and obstetrics work as a team to accomplish clinical duties, and both attend educational opportunities sponsored by the Department of Obstetrics and Gynecology.

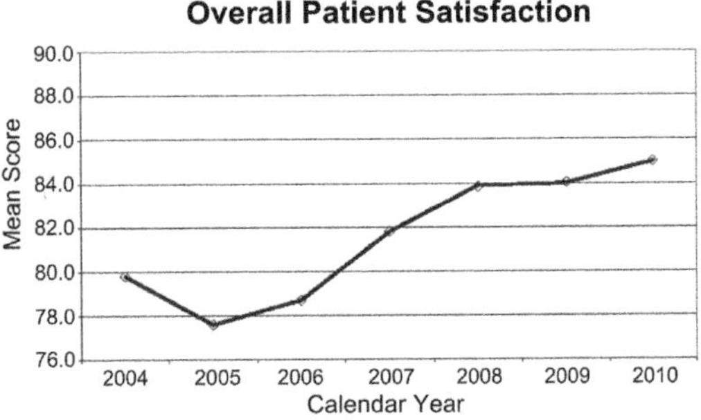


**Fig. 4.** Press Ganey scores from 2004 to 2010.

The chief resident serves as the consultant for the midwife with obstetrician back-up, providing opportunity to learn consultation skills for future practice.

Midwives are involved in many aspects of the obstetrics and gynecology residency program, including interviewing applicants, orientation, didactic, and clinical teaching. Didactic teaching includes a workshop on labor and delivery skills, a lecture on the evidence-based practices in the management of normal labor and birth and a workshop for chief residents on the role of the consultant in collaborative maternity care. In 2010, midwives initiated teaching midwifery students for the first time since the institution of the collaborative model. Midwifery students benefit from learning to work in an interdisciplinary collaborative environment and develop skills on interprofessional communication, which will be crucial for midwives in the coming decades. Midwifery students will be involved in educational programs of the 3 disciplines represented on labor and delivery and will give presentations on topics related to the management of normal childbirth. The involvement of midwives in medical education[38] is growing throughout the country, and interdisciplinary education has been noted as a potential ingredient in effective collaborative practice.[26]

Residents of family medicine and obstetrics now work daily with family physicians and midwives who provide maternity care. This model may improve the willingness of obstetrics graduates to collaborate with family physicians[39] and midwives in their future practices and address workforce issues in our communities.[38,39] Enhanced role modeling, patient-centered care, and early exposure to labor and delivery may encourage more family medicine residents to include maternity care in their future practices.[40,41]

Interdisciplinary education in the outpatient setting has expanded because of the inpatient collaboration between departments. Obstetrics residents rotate in family medicine clinics and family medicine residents rotate in obstetrics and gynecology clinics. Midwives are the cornerstone of resident education in group prenatal visits. A midwife-family physician team introduced group prenatal care using the Centering Pregnancy model[42] at 2 community health centers where residents of family medicine care for their continuity patients. This team plans to expand group prenatal care at additional health centers.

Obstetrics and family medicine residents respect and appreciate teaching from midwives and family physicians as a result of our collaborative model. Three years ago, the obstetrics residents created separate teaching awards for midwives and family physicians in addition to the teaching award given to their own faculty member. In 2009, the family medicine residents presented a midwife with the annual family medicine teaching award.

## SUMMARY

An invitation for more volume and revenue, 3 disciplines with respect for each other at the leadership level, and support from the hospital to address patient safety, enabled us to change the culture of the labor and delivery unit. For years, individuals practiced alongside each other in silos with variable interaction and respect for one another. Now, individuals come together to provide care as a true team. Communication occurs frequently among different provider types, nurses, obstetrics, and family medicine residents. Hierarchy is de-emphasized. Patient workloads are distributed equitably with thoughtful consideration of each patient's medical, social, and cultural needs. Workload distribution resulted in improving and maintaining the skills of family physicians. Through this culture of collaboration the authors' have optimized interdisciplinary education, which has been shown to improve patient outcomes and increase respect among those involved.

## ACKNOWLEDGMENTS

Brian Jack, MD, Susanna Erber, MD, Catherine Walker, CNM, MPH, Mayra Mieses for their work in design and implementation of this model and for contributing to this manuscript.

## REFERENCES

1. Anderson BL, Hale RW, Salsberg E, et al. Outlook for the future of the obstetrician-gynecologist workforce. Am J Obstet Gynecol 2008;199(1):88.e81–8.
2. Bettes BA, Chalas E, Coleman VH, et al. Heavier workload, less personal control: impact of delivery on obstetrician/gynecologists' career satisfaction. Am J Obstet Gynecol 2004;190(3):851–7.
3. Dresden GM, Baldwin LM, Andrilla CH, et al. Influence of obstetric practice on workload and practice patterns of family physicians and obstetrician-gynecologists. Ann Fam Med 2008;6(Suppl 1):S5–11.
4. Hueston WJ, Applegate JA, Mansfield CJ, et al. Practice variations between family physicians and obstetricians in the management of low-risk pregnancies. J Fam Pract 1995;40(4):345–51.
5. Coco AS, Gates TJ, Gallagher ME, et al. Association of attending physician specialty with the cesarean delivery rate in the same patient population. Fam Med 2000;32(9):639–44.
6. Hueston WJ, Lewis-Stevenson S. Provider distribution and variations in statewide cesarean section rates. J Community Health 2001;26(1):1–10.
7. Hatem M, Sandall J, Devane D, et al. Midwife-led versus other models of care for childbearing women. Cochrane Database Syst Rev 2008;(4):CD004667.
8. Hueston WJ, Rudy M. A comparison of labor and delivery management between nurse midwives and family physicians. J Fam Pract 1993;37(5):449–54.
9. MacDorman MF, Singh GK. Midwifery care, social and medical risk factors, and birth outcomes in the USA. J Epidemiol Community Health 1998;52(5):310–7.
10. Oakley D, Murray ME, Murtland T, et al. Comparisons of outcomes of maternity care by obstetricians and certified nurse-midwives. Obstet Gynecol 1996;88(5):823–9.
11. Rosenblatt RA, Dobie SA, Hart LG, et al. Interspecialty differences in the obstetric care of low-risk women. Am J Public Health 1997;87(3):344–51.
12. Turnbull D, Holmes A, Shields N, et al. Randomised, controlled trial of efficacy of midwife-managed care. Lancet 1996;348(9022):213–8.
13. Butler J, Abrams B, Parker J, et al. Supportive nurse-midwife care is associated with a reduced incidence of cesarean section. Am J Obstet Gynecol 1993;168(5):1407–13.
14. Chang Pecci C, Leeman L, Wilkinson J. Family medicine obstetrics fellowship graduates: training and post-fellowship experience. Fam Med 2008;40(5):326–32.
15. Rodney WM, Martinez C, Collins M, et al. OB fellowship outcomes 1992-2010: where do they go, who stops delivering, and why? Fam Med 2010;42(10):712–6.
16. Peterson WE, Medves JM, Davies BL, et al. Multidisciplinary collaborative maternity care in Canada: easier said than done. J Obstet Gynaecol Can 2007;29(11):880–6.
17. American College of Nurse-Midwives, American College of Obstetricians and Gynecologists. Joint statement of practice relations between obstetrician-gynecologists and certified nurse-midwives/certified midwives. Washington, DC: American College of Obstetricians and Gynecologists; 2011. Available at: http://bit.ly/iPoxJ3.

18. AAFP–ACOG joint statement of cooperative practice and hospital privileges. American Academy of Family Physicians. American College of Obstetricians and Gynecologists. Am Fam Physician 1998;58(1):277–8.
19. Nusbaum MR, Helton MR. A birth crisis. Fam Med 2002;34(6):423–5.
20. Veltman LL. Disruptive behavior in obstetrics: a hidden threat to patient safety. Am J Obstet Gynecol 2007;196(6):587. e581–4; [discussion: 587.e584–5].
21. Youngson R, Wimbrow T, Stacey T. A crisis in maternity services: the courage to be wrong. Qual Saf Health Care 2003;12(6):398–400.
22. Downe S, Finlayson K, Fleming A. Creating a collaborative culture in maternity care. J Midwifery Womens Health 2010;55(3):250–4.
23. Keleher KC. Collaborative practice. Characteristics, barriers, benefits, and implications for midwifery. J Nurse Midwifery 1998;43(1):8–11.
24. Reiger KM, Lane KL. Working together: collaboration between midwives and doctors in public hospitals. Aust Health Rev 2009;33(2):315–24.
25. Pinki P, Sayasneh A, Lindow SW. The working relationship between midwives and junior doctors: a questionnaire survey of Yorkshire trainees. J Obstet Gynaecol 2007;27(4):365–7.
26. Saxell L, Harris S, Elarar L. The Collaboration for Maternal and Newborn Health: interprofessional maternity care education for medical, midwifery, and nursing students. J Midwifery Womens Health 2009;54(4):314–20.
27. Singleton JK, Green-Hernandez C. Interdisciplinary education and practice. Has its time come? J Nurse Midwifery 1998;43(1):3–7.
28. Berridge EJ, Mackintosh NJ, Freeth DS. Supporting patient safety: examining communication within delivery suite teams through contrasting approaches to research observation. Midwifery 2010;26(5):512–9.
29. Harris KT, Treanor CM, Salisbury ML. Improving patient safety with team coordination: challenges and strategies of implementation. J Obstet Gynecol Neonatal Nurs 2006;35(4):557–66.
30. Leape LL. Scope of problem and history of patient safety. Obstet Gynecol Clin North Am 2008;35(1):1–10, vii.
31. Lemieux-Charles L, McGuire WL. What do we know about health care team effectiveness? A review of the literature. Med Care Res Rev 2006;63(3):263–300.
32. Pratt SD, Mann S, Salisbury M, et al. John M. Eisenberg Patient Safety and Quality Awards. Impact of CRM-based training on obstetric outcomes and clinicians' patient safety attitudes. Jt Comm J Qual Patient Saf 2007;33(12):720–5.
33. Smith AH, Dixon AL, Page LA. Health-care professionals' views about safety in maternity services: a qualitative study. Midwifery 2009;25(1):21–31.
34. American College of Obstetricians and Gynecologists Committee Committee on Patient Safety and Quality Improvement. ACOG Committee Opinion No. 447: patient safety in obstetrics and gynecology. Obstet Gynecol 2009;114(6):1424–7. DOI:1410.1097/AOG.1420b1013e3181c1426f1490e.
35. King H, Battles J, Baker D, et al. TeamSTEPPS™: team strategies and tools to enhance performance and patient safety. Department of Defense and the Agency for Healthcare Research and Quality. Rockville (MD): Agency for Healthcare Research and Quality; 2006.
36. Skinner JP, Foureur M. Consultation, referral, and collaboration between midwives and obstetricians: lessons from New Zealand. J Midwifery Womens Health 2010;55(1):28–37.
37. Iverson RE Jr, Heffner LJ. Obstetric safety improvement and its reflection in reserved claims. Am J Obstet Gynecol 2011;205(5):398–401.

38. McConaughey E, Howard E. Midwives as educators of medical students and residents: results of a national survey. J Midwifery Womens Health 2009;54(4): 268–74.
39. Topping DB, Hueston WJ, MacGilvray P. Family physicians delivering babies: what do obstetricians think? Fam Med 2003;35(10):737–41.
40. Larimore WL, Reynolds JL. Family practice maternity care in America: ruminations on reproducing an endangered species–family physicians who deliver babies. J Am Board Fam Pract 1994;7(6):478–88.
41. Ratcliffe SD, Newman SR, Stone MB, et al. Obstetric care in family practice residencies: a 5-year follow-up survey. J Am Board Fam Pract 2002;15(1):20–4.
42. Manant A, Dodgson JE. CenteringPregnancy: an integrative literature review. J Midwifery Womens Health 2011;56(2):94–102.

# Midwifery and Obstetrics

## Twenty Years of Collaborative Academic Practice

Diane J. Angelini, EdD, CNM[a,b,*], Barbara O'Brien, MD[b,c], Janet Singer, MSN, CNM[b,c], Donald R. Coustan, MD[b,c]

**KEYWORDS**

• Obstetrics • Midwifery • Residents • Medical students • Partnering

**KEY POINTS**

- This article describes a 20-year successful and collaborative academic practice between obstetrics and midwifery in the education of obstetric residents and medical students.
- This model highlights resident education by midwives primarily in low-risk obstetrics and within an obstetric triage and emergency setting.
- Midwives involved in medical education are in a pivotal position to have an impact on the education on the next generation of obstetricians and consultants.

Midwives have been actively involved in medical education since the 1980s and possibly earlier.[1] The incorporation of midwifery faculty in the education of medical students and residents, however, has grown exponentially over the past 20 years.[2–7] A 1998 survey of midwives involved in medical education noted that more than half of the allopathic medical school clerkships in obstetrics and gynecology (OB/GYN) used midwives as educators in the United States.[6] Approximately 10 years later that rate had tripled.[7] A companion survey of academic midwifery directors involved in medical education across the United States documented the key leadership role of the midwifery director in achieving these outcomes.[8]

The growth of these models coincides with a decrease in resident work hours and increasing demand for interprofessional educational collaboration.[9] Both an interprofessional approach and collaborative efforts are required for the success of such teaching models and the means to eliminating practice barriers.[10–12] Interprofessional implies professions working together in collaboration by integrating services and using teamwork concepts, eliminating the silo effect. This article (1) details a collaborative

No funding sources.

[a] Nurse Midwifery Section, Women & Infants Hospital of Rhode Island, Alpert Medical School of Brown University, 101 Dudley Street, Providence, RI 02905, USA; [b] Department of Obstetrics and Gynecology, Alpert Medical School of Brown University, 101 Dudley Street, Providence, RI 02905, USA; [c] Women & Infants Hospital of Rhode Island, Alpert Medical School of Brown University, 101 Dudley Street, Providence, RI 02905, USA

* Corresponding author.

*E-mail address:* dangelini@wihri.org

Obstet Gynecol Clin N Am 39 (2012) 335–346

http://dx.doi.org/10.1016/j.ogc.2012.05.002 obgyn.theclinics.com

0889-8545/12/$ – see front matter 

practice of midwives integrated into medical education in a department of OB/GYN, which developed over 20 years; (2) highlights evaluative data and productivity; and (3) addresses teaching efforts, specifically in labor and birth, as well as in the obstetric triage/emergency setting.

## COLLABORATION

Collaboration is a dynamic, flexible nonhierarchical process involving the efforts of more than one person to accomplish a mutually determined goal.[12] Individual skills, strengths, and limitations are combined into one collaborative mix. Levels of authority may rise and fall for each member[13] because collaboration reflects a give-and-take process in the context of changing power balances.[14–17] Collaboration is generally a shared dynamic function requiring the will to make meaningful contact and respect the extent and limits of each individual's skills when professionals gather in a clinical environment for education and training purposes.[12]

The collaborative model involves 2 levels of behavior: those reflected in an individual's skill set and those shown by the team as a whole.[18] Collaboration is accomplished through an environment of mutual respect, good communication, and trust. The comanagement of care through the collaborative model, as described by Keleher,[17] relies on smooth integration of team members so that members can work together to accomplish a task that neither could accomplish alone.

As artificial reproductive technologies, medical technologies, and survival rates of many diseases advance, many more women with complex medical disorders are achieving pregnancies. Although more complex medically, some of their fundamental educational and psychosocial needs are typical of those for any pregnant woman.[18] Collaboration between midwives and physicians provides an opportunity for select medically complex patients to continue with midwifery care with OB/GYN physician consultation, as needed. Among other skills, midwifery expertise includes the management of normal pregnancies and social and psychological issues as well as recognition of deviation from the norm. Increasing collaboration between midwifery and medicine allows more complex medical patients the benefits of both disciplines. This is particularly valuable where rapid transfer between care providers may become necessary.[12] The model also allows for a greater number of patients to be cared for in a team approach, allocating attending obstetricians to address more complex cases.

## BACKGROUND

In 1990, a collaborative effort between the Women & Infants Hospital of Rhode Island and the Department of Obstetrics and Gynecology at the Alpert Medical School of Brown University was undertaken to establish an academic, educational practice model where midwives became part of the teaching faculty for medical students and residents. Although medical students and residents are the primary customers in this education model, women and their infants are the ultimate beneficiaries. The midwifery section was established within the Department of Obstetrics and Gynecology in 1990 with a direct reporting mechanism of the midwifery director to the chairperson of OB/GYN.

The addition of midwives to the medical faculty in 1990 was intended to fill several needs. A busy resident service did not allow adequate or quality teaching time or elective opportunities. A higher proportion of resident time was spent on service needs and not on improving resident education needs. This threatened the quality of the residency. At this same time, the medical student clerkship was poorly rated and residents did not have adequate time to teach. There was no clear systematic approach to resident education in basic obstetrics and limited feedback was provided.

To address these problems, experienced midwives were hired to serve as additional clinical teachers for the low-risk obstetric resident practice in a collaborative, team approach in collaboration with attending obstetricians. A noncompetitive model was established with residents and medical students where the caseload was cared for by all. This has been termed, a fully integrated model,[19] in which the midwives act as a member of the resident team without a separate private practice. The model's strength is in its demonstration of collaborative practice with enhanced communication among residents, midwifery faculty, and attending obstetricians. The midwifery philosophy and the medical model intersect at the point of care. Attending obstetricians in this model are available to the midwives for consultation and backup. They also are freed up to teach operative obstetrics, comanage cesarean births with residents, and manage selected high-risk cases. The model for attending staff consists of more than 100 hospital and community obstetricians who rotate in 4 teams, each team taking 1 month on service.

Additional clinical opportunities and the need to expand teaching into the first 2 years of the residency allowed the midwives to broaden their teaching focus early in the development of this model. More curriculum-based and-in-depth teaching of postgraduate year (PGY) 1 and PGY2 residents in labor/birth and obstetric triage resulted in an overall expansion of midwifery services and direct input and incorporation into the curriculum of the residency.

## PRACTICE MODEL AND SETTING

The practice site for this model is a stand-alone hospital, specializing in women's health and neonatal care, affiliated with the Alpert Medical School of Brown University. It has a history of a busy obstetric service from just under 10,000 births in 1990 to 8528 births in fiscal year 2010.[20] It is the only tertiary-level center for obstetrics and neonatal care in Rhode Island and is a primary referral hospital for southeastern New England. More than 73% of Rhode Island births occur in this setting; 25% are attended by obstetric residents.

The population served by the resident practice includes a catchment area principally in central and south Providence, Rhode Island, and from health centers throughout the city. Parts of this catchment area qualify for National Health Service Corps loan repayment because many parts of Rhode Island, including Providence are designated health professional shortage areas.[21] Most of the women cared for by the resident service are considered vulnerable because they are medically underserved and many are poor.[22] At the hospital site, women receive prenatal care from nurse practitioners and residents. In the health centers, obstetricians and advanced practice nurses provide prenatal and gynecologic services. Births for both hospital and health center patients are attended at the women's hospital by residents, midwives, and attending obstetricians in the Department of Obstetrics and Gynecology.

Before 1990, no midwives were employed in the Department of Obstetrics and Gynecology. The first midwife was recruited in 1990 as director to develop the program working with the resident intrapartum caseload. As of 2010 there are 6 full-time equivalents for midwifery faculty.

A critical element in the success of this model is that midwives do not have a private caseload of patients. Sharing a common caseload with obstetric residents is a unique model of midwifery clinical practice.[19] It has brought residents, midwives, and attending obstetricians closer, however, in their dialogue about clinical management decisions by reducing the competitive issues and contrasting viewpoints. The authors believe this provides for a more collaborative approach and a mutually respectful relationship.

## MEDICAL STUDENT EDUCATION

In 1992, with support from the director of medical education, the midwives assumed responsibility for medical student education during the students' 2-week labor and delivery rotation, teaching approximately 3 to 4 students every 2 weeks. Formal classes on basic labor care and management, fetal assessment, and hand skills for birth were developed and implemented. Principles of suturing, dexterity with surgical instruments, and laceration repair were taught and midwives attended births with medical students. Along with the shift to a skills emphasis in the medical school curriculum, objective structured clinical examinations (OSCEs) were implemented in the form of simulation stations to assess core competencies of students during the obstetric clerkship.[23] This shift marked a critical turning point in the integration of midwifery into the Department of Obstetrics and Gynecology teaching program. The midwives taught skills and clinical assessment to the students and participated in the simulated scenarios used to assess competency. This effort is coordinated by one midwifery faculty member who coordinates medical student instruction in obstetrics in collaboration with the core clerkship director and has been highly successful.

## RESIDENT EDUCATION

In 1994, the midwives increased their involvement with resident teaching in response to increasing demands for instruction of PGY1 and PGY2 residents in low-risk obstetrics. From 1994 to the present, midwives have remained actively involved in resident learning in labor/birth and obstetric triage. The role of the midwifery practice stretched across the PGY1 and PGY2 years to ultimately have input into all 4 years of resident training while showcasing collaborative practice between midwifery and physician faculties.

Midwives lead the resident boot camp training in clinical skills with a heavy reliance on simulation to enhance the PGY1 resident competency in conjunction with other faculty during the orientation week held each June. The curricula taught by midwives, based on clinical content skills and simulated learning sessions, validate competency and identify any needed remediation (**Table 1**).

## THE MODEL IN ACTION: LABOR AND BIRTH

The team for the low-risk resident practice on the labor unit consists of a chief resident, a PGY1 resident, a PGY2 resident, a midwife, 3 to 4 medical students, and an attending physician for consultation and backup in the management of complex obstetric complications. Decisions on labor management are shared among all team members for normal and problematic labors. Clinical decision making is viewed as a collaborative academic dialogue in which the midwifery perspective and the medical perspective are considered and weighed together. This approach engenders respect for the mutual contributions of all parties and has become an effective teaching modality for the education of residents, which supports dimensions of collaborative practice.

Respect for others is a specific focus in this collaborative model. Experienced midwives model how to approach and speak to patients; this has assisted new physicians in training to develop and hone similar communicative styles. Midwives and attending obstetricians demonstrate the value of mutual respect within the team concept, allowing for openness, collaboration, and true partnership. Although the

**Table 1**
**Specific teaching curricula and clinical skill development for obstetric residents**

| | Resident Level | |
|---|---|---|
| **Curricula** | **PGY 1** | **PGY 2** |
| Labor and birth | • Vaginal examinations<br>• Amniotomy<br>• Hand maneuvers for birth<br>• Suturing and laceration repair<br>• Basic fetal heart rate monitoring/interpretation<br>• Clinical management of postpartum hemorrhage and shoulder dystocia | • Refinement of vaginal examinations (including clinical pelvimetry)<br>• Advanced labor management<br>• Pain management therapies<br>• Advanced suturing and laceration repair<br>• Intrapartum fetal resuscitation<br>• Complications review: postpartum hemorrhage, shoulder dystocia, uterine inversion, preeclampsia/eclampsia |
| Obstetric triage/emergency care | • Speculum/vaginal examinations<br>• Fetal assessment<br>• Limited ultrasound<br>• Use of labor induction agents<br>• Labor evaluation<br>• Nausea/vomiting of pregnancy<br>• Clinical complications >20 weeks' gestation<br>○ Decreased fetal movement<br>○ Noncatastrophic trauma<br>○ Preeclampsia/gestational hypertension<br>○ Urinary tract infection<br>○ Vaginal bleeding<br>○ Preterm labor<br>○ Preterm premature rupture of membranes<br>○ Abdominal pain | Continued consultation for PGY2 residents with clinical complications >20 weeks' gestation |

benefits to this collaborative model have been refined over many years and advance with each new resident class, its value lies in having multiple perspectives brought to each clinical encounter. Such an integrated practice model supports the concept that midwifery and obstetrics can partner together to improve both educational outcomes and interprofessional, collaborative clinical teaching.

## CREDENTIALING AND DIRECT SUPERVISION

Each PGY1 resident attends 20 to 30 births with a midwife, in addition to rotations in the operating room, postpartum rounds, and obstetric triage. Expected communication skills at the end of the rotation include the ability to "handle the birthing room" (ie, managing the birth itself, assessing the fetus, and work with nursing staff, family members, and other medical personnel). The ability to move away from focusing on the perineum, toward addressing the complete needs of the woman and infant, as well as managing any complications, is the overall goal of the curriculum at this level.

This clinical competency is now well integrated into the overall model, and it is viewed by residents as a rite of passage when they are permitted to attend births alone. A key to the effectiveness of this model is the chief resident of obstetrics who supports the model and expects to know when PGY1 can be assessed as competent to attend a birth independently. This model has developed over years to reach this level of give and take, mutual respect, and accepted expectations.

In addition to the PGY1 resident, the PGY2 resident is a critical member of the low-risk obstetric team on the labor unit. Midwifery faculty undertook responsibility for the education of the PGY2 residents in labor and delivery. Specific teaching curricula and clinical skill development are listed in **Table 1**.

## OBSTETRIC TRIAGE AND EMERGENT CARE

The concept of obstetric triage is well documented in the literature, and triage concepts are now fully integrated into obstetric services for pregnant women.[24–26] The annual number of obstetric visits in triage/emergency care at Women & Infants Hospital of Rhode Island in fiscal year 2010 was 27,903,[20] with approximately 73% obstetric related, most (62%) greater than 20 weeks' gestation. Midwifery faculty and a separate group of triage/emergency obstetricians instruct residents in this setting. This has broadened the development and use of midwives and obstetricians who can teach residents new skill sets, clinical evidence–based guidelines, and management skills in an obstetric emergency setting.[25]

The academic midwives and obstetricians in the triage setting provide for a smooth transition for residents new to their role as well as a safety net in a setting that requires quick decision making, rapid turnover, and multiple handoffs. The competency format for PGY1 residents used in this rotation is listed in **Table 1**. Basic ultrasound skills are incorporated as part of a 4-year learning ultrasound curriculum, which enables residents to use ultrasound data to complete full management of each case and sets the groundwork for eventual ultrasound certification.

As PGY1 residents attain competency in this setting, they are eventually permitted to evaluate patients alone with consultation only. Faculty members, however, assess all patients who are evaluated by residents, review fetal tracings, and bill for appropriate services. The physician staff members in triage assume care for pregnant women less than 20 weeks' gestation and women with significant gynecologic conditions and complex medical issues. They are responsible for all resident teaching efforts (PGY1–PGY4). Both physician attending staff and midwifery faculty work collaboratively in this unit in a team approach to patient care and resident teaching.

## ADDITIONAL PRACTICE DIMENSIONS AND INNOVATIONS

With decreases in resident work hours and improvements in reimbursement and billing opportunities, midwives have seen expansion of their practice and added value to the department as faculty. Additional responsibilities assumed by the midwives include serving as first assistants on cesarean births and initiation of postpartum rounding on uncomplicated postpartum women. Expansion to evening hours in the triage setting has assisted residents in completing competency requirements and provides additional billing and revenue opportunities for midwives.

## DEPARTMENTAL STRUCTURE

As with any program that has been sustained for 20 years, active representation on hospital and departmental committees is vital. Key representation by midwifery faculty includes resident evaluation, graduate medical education, and promotions and credentials committees; core clerkship meetings; and the educational council, where the faculty members responsible for medical education discuss strategic planning and educational goals. Midwives also meet monthly with the residency directors and the medical director of triage to improve on collaborative and communicative efforts relative to resident teaching in labor and triage settings. A faculty midwife also sits on the obstetric review committee. Midwives also qualify for faculty appointments in the school of medicine using promotion criteria required of all faculty members, including promotion to full clinical professor, recently achieved by one member.

Collaboration across divisions within the Department of Obstetrics and Gynecology has been crucial for academic midwifery to gain credibility among faculty peers. One of the long-standing simulation workshops in existence within the Department of Obstetrics and Gynecology is on suturing and advanced laceration repair offered jointly by midwifery and urogynecology faculty for ascending PGY3 residents. Other simulation learning experiences include a day-long PGY1 orientation workshop boot camp, an advanced skills workshop for PGY2 residents, and a leadership workshop for PGY4 residents as they transition into their last year.[27] The leadership workshop builds on Synectics, a creative problem-solving technique[28,29] used by Fortune 500 companies. This technique allows for new connections and ideas to be identified in a creative fashion to solve problems. The midwives meet with each chief resident as they begin their rotation as chief of low-risk obstetrics, refreshing the conversation about leadership.

## MENTORING

A mentoring program for new residents was initiated in 1996. This is one of many innovations within this collaborative educational practice model (**Table 2**). The mentoring program links residents with midwifery faculty in the first year. Initially, each midwife is assigned to 1 or 2 newly matched residents, who are contacted by e-mail before their arrival for orientation. The midwives have already met them during their interviews for the residency, so this links them together early in that first and significant year of education. The mentoring eases the transition and provides a solid support base for each PGY1 resident, from medical student to first-year resident, providing a safety net for issues arising during the first year. Midwives transition the residents to both a hospital-based faculty and a community-based faculty to ensure each resident has 2 physician mentors after the completion of the first year of residency.

## STATE REGULATORY AND CREDENTIALING ISSUES

State regulations can exert significant impact on midwifery practice.[29] The State of Rhode Island has separate provision for rules and regulations that address the licensing of midwives, which provide for an advisory council, prescriptive privileges, disciplinary action, and continuing education requirements for midwives. Within the Women & Infants Hospital of Rhode Island, the credentialing of midwives occurs through the credentials committee, which includes a midwife representative. Midwives are credentialed as allied health professionals within the hospital bylaws and can bill for services but do not have admitting privileges.

## OUTCOMES

A variety of educational interventions, reflected in different evaluative data outcomes, have been achieved in this model. Data from teaching evaluations, exit interviews with

**Table 2**
**Model innovations and collaborative efforts**

| Innovation | Value-Added Benefits and Collaborative Efforts |
|---|---|
| Noncompetitive model | • Limits competition among providers<br>• Focuses on learner<br>• Decreases conflict among all collaborators |
| Obstetric triage/emergency component | • Increases collaboration with triage/ emergency attending obstetricians<br>• Added teaching site<br>• Additional revenue source<br>• Midwives act as safety net for resident handoffs |
| Mentoring program | • Strong resident/midwife linkage established early in residency<br>• Mechanism for sustained resident contact with physician faculty throughout residency |
| Meetings with chief residents each obstetric rotation | • Renews linkage among midwives, residents, and faculty<br>• Refreshes leadership conversation and prior linkage with leadership workshop |
| Clinical competency programs | • Specific skills and teaching developed for PGY1 in labor and delivery/obstetric triage and for PGY2 in labor and delivery |
| Collaboration across departmental divisions | • Access for collaborative research<br>• Linkage for collaborative simulation training and education |
| Simulation learning experiences and workshops | • ↑ Teaching exposure of faculty<br>• Demonstrates additional, in-depth teaching capabilities<br>• ↑ Interdepartmental collaboration across academic divisions |
| Faculty appointments in medical school | • Parity with other faculty |

chief residents, and research achievements of the midwifery faculty over the past 20 years are discussed in this section.

In the 20 years that the midwifery faculty have been contributing to medical education, they have taught a total of 1478 medical students and 168 OB/GYN residents and have received numerous teaching and other recognition awards. On a 5-point Likert scale (5 being the highest score) from 5 years' worth of data (2005–2010), midwifery teaching scores were uniformly favorably evaluated, with mean scores of 4.68 from residents and 4.46 from medical students. Three midwifery faculty members ranked in the top 13% of 114 total faculty members based on electronic resident evaluations from 2005 to 2010.

Qualitative data analysis of online evaluations by medical students identified specific categories of what students valued most about the midwifery faculty, including advocacy, feedback, and skills building. Students valued the midwives for seeking out learning experiences for them, serving as advocates for their learning, providing valuable feedback, and teaching practical skills. Medical students described the midwives as passionate and patient teachers who are invested in medical education.

Qualitative data analysis of online evaluations by residents of midwifery faculty identified excellence across the following themes: support, feedback, perspective, and knowledge. Residents valued the support the midwives provide, describing them as "surrogate moms," "a calm presence," and "an advocate." They particularly appreciate the valuable, timely, and constructive feedback the midwives provide, indicated by "lets me know areas I needed to work on" and "fosters clinical and personal growth." Residents emphasized that the teaching they receive from the midwives is different from what they receive from other faculty members—describing the midwives as "a voice for creativity and thinking outside the box," "humanistic," and "offers a different perspective."

A 5-year (2005–2010) summary of evaluative data from 4 simulation workshops taught by midwives showed a mean score of 4.91 of 5 on a Likert scale and median score of 4.94 of 5. Qualitative statements from residents illuminate the changing relationship the residents have with the midwives, as they progress from year to year. After spending a day during PGY1 orientation in the skills workshop, known as intern boot camp, the interns reveal their anxiety/fear and are extremely appreciative: "so open and helpful with our questions"; "I feel much more comfortable about starting now"; "Thank you for assuming we know nothing"; and "You made me feel more confident." Approaching their fourth and final year, the residents once again feel trepidation and appreciate getting to explore their new chief role with the midwives in the leadership workshop: "I think I am ready…what a great rite of passage"; "I'm glad to know that I am not alone in all my fears"; and "Gave me confidence for next year."

In exit interview data, residents commented, "This residency would not be what it is without the midwives" and "God forbid the midwives should ever leave this place." When chief residents were asked to name 3 strengths of the residency program in exit interviews, the midwives and patient volume were mentioned more than any other attribute over the 4 years, 2007 through 2010 (unpublished data from Gary Frishman, MD, personal communication, 2010).

The midwifery faculty members have also been productive scholars. Research endeavors over the 20 years by the midwifery faculty total 32 peer-reviewed articles, 3 books, and 16 book chapters. Seventy-six national and international posters/abstracts and 94 local, national, and international presentations have been presented.

## CHALLENGES

Significant barriers have been encountered in implementing this collaborative educational model. First, the obstetrics residents had not previously worked with midwives before 1990. Making decisions about patient care in a collaborative fashion was new. Early on, experienced midwives had to prove their clinical acumen and often assumed the role of novice in a new model. Working with more than 100 hospital-based and community-based faculty members who served as consultants was difficult. Every day there was a different attending physician, many of whom had never worked with midwives or had negative past experiences with midwives. The key challenge for the midwife was to establish mutual respect and trust at the point of care. Managing births together with residents and attending physicians over time provided the linchpin for respect between midwife and resident as well as between midwife and attending physician.

The institutional financial support for midwives, without a private caseload of patients, was possible in return for improvements in teaching and liberating residents to pursue needed educational experiences. Midwives do forecast productivity statistics year-to-year and generate revenue from services in obstetric triage and postpartum rounds.

**Box 1**
**Key components of midwifery model**

- Direct reporting mechanism to the chairperson of OB/GYN
- Champions for midwifery developed among physician faculty
- Hospital and institutional support from initiation of program
- Key midwifery leaders recruited in early establishment of model
- Midwifery faculty with specific teaching skills recruited to advance clinical teaching model

No process that sustains itself for 20 years does so without champions and supportive partners.[8] The chairperson of OB/GYN is key in this endeavor. Establishing the reporting mechanism early on of the midwifery director to the chairperson provided for direct access and support. In one survey, 66% of midwifery directors in an academic medical teaching setting reported to the chairperson.[8] This seems to be a successful national trend and has been used in this model for 20 years. The directors of the residency and core clerkship have been crucial advocates to the success of this collaborative model and they include midwifery faculty in decision making at all levels. Academic and clinical appointments for the midwifery faculty are championed by the departmental chairperson. The inclusion of midwives in key committees, such as promotions and credentials, helps support midwifery in the department and within the institution. Advocating for inclusion and using key faculty to support midwifery involvement in hospital-wide committees are integral to success.

## MODEL REPLICATION

This collaborative educational model has attracted national and international visitors seeking input as they contemplate a new paradigm of medical education in their own institutions as well as other midwives, residency directors, and medical faculty visiting during the 20 years of this model's existence. Key components of successful replication of this model are listed in **Box 1**.

The triage/emergency component is innovative to this institution and educational model and has become the basis for other triage models across the country.[25] It has been a financial strength for the midwives who are able to bill for services in triage while teaching residents and working collaboratively with triage attending physicians, including the medical director, who must be a strong supporter of midwifery.

## FUTURE INITIATIVES

Future changes in resident work hours would have a direct impact on midwifery faculty in an interdisciplinary model where resident education is dominant. This can be viewed positively but may also dilute midwives' ability to produce positive results if midwifery is used to fill service gaps and not balanced with time for educational responsibilities. Aspects of future direction for the educational ventures of this model include instituting a more interdisciplinary model for postpartum rounds and expanding opportunities for simulated teaching experiences in a new simulation center in collaboration with other academic faculty.

## SUMMARY

This noncompetitive, integrated educational practice model has been a successful and collaborative effort between obstetrics and midwifery using midwives as clinical faculty within an academic department of OB/GYN. The model highlights resident teaching by midwives primarily in low-risk obstetrics in collaboration with attending obstetricians in the labor unit and in the obstetric triage/emergency setting. Midwives involved in medical education are in a pivotal position to have an impact on the education of the next generation of obstetricians and consultants while showcasing the midwifery model of care. This opens the door to the future of collaborative practice through innovation in OB/GYN residency education.

## REFERENCES

1. Platt L, Angelini D, Paul R, et al. Nurse midwifery in a large teaching hospital. Obstet Gynecol 1985;66:816–20.
2. Metheny W, Angelini D. Successful integration of midwifery into an academic department of Ob/Gyn. Ann Behav Sci Med Educ 2000;7:39–44.
3. Sedler K, Lyndon-Rochelle M, Castillo Y, et al. Nurse midwifery service model in an academic environment. J Nurse Midwifery 1993;38:241–5.
4. Fineland J, Sankey TR. The obstetric team: midwives teaching residents and medical students on the labor and delivery unit. J Midwifery Womens Health 2008;53:376–80.
5. Mankoff R, DeVore N, Freda M. Orientation of OB GYN residents to ambulatory care: a nurse midwifery approach. J Nurse Midwifery 1994;39:375–8.
6. Harman P, Summers L, King T, et al. Interdisciplinary teaching: a survey of CNM participation in medical education in the United States. J Nurse Midwifery 1998;43:27–35.
7. McConaughey E, Howard E. Midwives as educators of medical students and residents: results of a national survey. J Midwifery Womens Health 2009;54:268–74.
8. Angelini D. A national survey of the midwifery director role in academic midwifery practices involved in medical education in the United States. J Midwifery Womens Health 2009;54:275–81.
9. Angelini D. Midwifery and medical education: a decade of changes [editorial]. J Midwifery Womens Health 2009;54:267.
10. Angelini D. The midwife's expanding role in interdisciplinary education. Proceedings from the Working Symposium on Midwifery. Canadian Conference of Midwives. Children's and Women's Health Centre of British Columbia. Vancouver, Canada, May 1-3, 2002. p. 91–7.
11. Tillett J. Nurses as interdisciplinary educators. J Perinat Neonatal Nurs 2007;21: 278–9.
12. Downe S, Finlayson K, Fleming A. Creating a collaborative culture in maternity care. J Midwifery Womens Health 2010;55:250–4.
13. Bailes A, Jackson M. Shared responsibility in home birth practice: collaborating with clients. J Midwifery Womens Health 2000;45:537–43.
14. Stichler J. Professional interdependence: the art of collaboration. Adv Pract Nurs Q 1995;1:53–61.
15. Stapleton S. Team building: making collaborative practice work. J Nurse Midwifery 1998;43:12–7.
16. Ivey SL, Brown KS, Teske Y, et al. A model for teaching about interdisciplinary practice in health care settings. J Allied Health 1998;17:189–95.
17. Keleher K. Collaborative practice: characteristics, barriers, benefits and implication for midwifery. J Nurse Midwifery 1998;43:8–11.
18. Gray M, D'Amato L. Medically complex pregnancy: a case report illustrating CNM/MD collaborative management. J Midwifery Womens Health 2000;45: 552–7.

19. Collins Fulea C. Models of organizational structure of midwifery practices located in institutions with residency programs. J Midwifery Womens Health 2009;54: 287–93.
20. Women and Infants Hospital of Rhode Island Annual Report. Providence (RI): Women and Infants Hospital of Rhode Island; 2010. p. 17.
21. U.S. Department of Health and Human Services. Health Resources and Service Administration (HRSA). Available at: http://bhpr.hrsa.gov/shortage/. Accessed November 22, 2010.
22. U.S. Department of Health and Human Services. Health Resources and Service Administration (HRSA). Available at: http://muafind.hrsa.gov/. Accessed November 22, 2010.
23. Department of Obstetrics and Gynecology Clerkship Program. Available at: http://brown.edu/Departments/ObstetricsGynecology/Clerkship.html. Accessed November 18, 2010.
24. Angelini D. The utilization of nurse midwives as providers of obstetric triage services. J Nurse Midwifery 1999;55:431–8.
25. Angelini D, Stevens E, MacDonald A, et al. Obstetric triage: models and trends in resident education by midwives. J Midwifery Womens Health 2009;54:294–300.
26. Ciranni P, Essex M. Better care, better bottom line: the impact of nurse practitioners in OB/GYN triage. Nurs Womens Health 2007;11:275–81.
27. Steinhardt L. Innovative midwifery teaching with residents. Brown University and Women & Infants Hospital. In Cooper E. Innovative Midwifery Teaching for Medical Students and Residents. J Midwifery Womens Health 2009;54:301–5.
28. Gordon W. Synectics: the development of creative capacity. New York: Harper; 1961.
29. Avery M, Germano E, Camune B. Midwifery practice and nursing regulation: licensure, accreditation, certification and education. J Midwifery Womens Health 2010;55:411–67.

# Description of a Successful Collaborative Birth Center Practice Among Midwives and an Obstetrician

Jennifer R. Stevens, CNM, MS[a,b,c,d,*],
Tammy L. Witmer, CNM, MSN[a,b,c,d], Robin L. Grant, CNM, MSN[a,b,c,d],
Dominic J. Cammarano III, DO[e,f]

**KEYWORDS**

• Midwifery • Obstetrics • Collaboration • Birth center • Maternity care

**KEY POINTS**

- Collaboration is the foundation of a successful birth center maternity care model to provide safe, individualized, high-quality, cost-effective care with good outcomes.
- Successful collaboration requires all members to be equally involved, valued and committed.
- Midwifery care model is optimized when allowed to function independently as a full member within the health care system utilizing collaboration.
- The birth center model provides the form and function for the full expression of midwifery care and engagement of the mother.

## INTRODUCTION

This article presents a birth center–based model as an ideal embodiment of collaborative care. The foundation of collaboration among an obstetrician-gynecologist (OB/GYN), a midwife, and the mother is the common goal of ensuring safe and satisfying care. Collaboration is defined by the 2011 Merriam-Webster online dictionary

[a] Reading Birth and Women's Center, 949 New Holland Road, Reading, PA 19607, USA; [b] American Association of Birth Centers, 3123 Gottschall Road, Reading, PA 18074, USA; [c] American College of Nurse Midwives, AABC 8403 Colesville Road, Suite 1550 Silver Spring, MD 20910, USA; [d] Commission for Accreditation of Birth Centers, 8345 NW 66th Street, # 6638 Miami, FL 33166, USA; [e] Reading OB/GYN and Women's Birth Center, 3701 Perkiomen Avenue, Reading, PA 19606, USA; [f] Section of Gynecology, Reading Hospital and Medical Center, Sixth and Spruce Street, Reading, PA 19611, USA

* Corresponding author. Reading OB/GYN and Women's Birth Center, 3701 Perkiomen Avenue, Reading, PA 19606.

*E-mail address:* RBWCjs@gmail.com

Obstet Gynecol Clin N Am 39 (2012) 347–357
http://dx.doi.org/10.1016/j.ogc.2012.05.003
obgyn.theclinics.com

as: "to work jointly with others or together especially in an intellectual endeavor."[1] Collaboration is optimal because it plays to each member's strengths. An OB/GYN is trained as a surgical specialist with a skill set needed for the surgical management of gynecologic and obstetric problems or complications that are outside a midwife's scope of practice. A midwife is educated in the normalcy of pregnancy and routine gynecologic care, and focuses on education and engaging the mother. The mother, who is the authority over her unique body and needs, is a vital part of the collaborative process. She communicates her needs and shares responsibility with her providers for a safe and satisfying outcome. A collaborative relationship, in which all feel equally valued, takes time to craft.

Collaborative practice is not a new concept in health care. Over the past 2 decades it has been packaged with different labels, including "nursing shared governance"[2] and "crew resource management" during obstetric emergency management, which replicates the team approach used in the airline industry.[3] Internationally, the collaborative practice model is well-known and addresses many of the current health care issues in the United States. Countries such as The Netherlands, Australia, New Zealand,[4] Sweden, and Canada[5] integrate collaborative practice models into their national health care structure, and their maternity care statistics provide compelling evidence that collaborative practice may contribute to success.

Most health care professionals would agree the United States is in a health care crisis, and the anticipated workforce shortage will only aggravate existing problems. As early as 1988, The Institute of Medicine's report on maternity care described the U.S. maternity care model as "fundamentally flawed, fragmented, and overly complex."[6] A report promoted by the Millbank Memorial Fund suggests the increased use of midwives and collaboration of care as a potential remedy to improve maternity care in the United States, where current outcomes in infant mortality are surprisingly poor and health care expenditures are high compared with other developed countries.[7–9] The report's systematic reviews of evidence focusing on maternity care suggested evidence-based solutions to the maternity care crisis. Research has shown that midwifery care is as safe as, and even more cost-effective than, traditional medically led care.[5,10] There is a current national and global call for health care reform.[11] Three of the eight World Health Organization's Millennium Development Goals 2010 address maternal child health. The final goal calls for a "global partnership," which implies collaboration.[12]

Another driving force in health care reform is the Internet-savvy health care consumer, who presents with complex issues and questions. Many consumers come prepared, having researched their concerns on the Internet, and expect a provider to help them to decipher the overabundance of information.[13] The traditional task-oriented model in which the provider has more power and control may not meet these consumers' needs. Many health care providers are recognizing this changing patient population and realizing that patients are expecting more from them. With this increased access to medical information and dissatisfaction with current care, a nationwide grassroots push exists for more midwifery-based care, as shown in Ricki Lake's 2008 documentary "The Business of Being Born."[14]

The authors' current collaborative practice model is grounded on the strong foundations and relationships built by an independent midwife and her collaborating physician. Although the original practice has grown and changed over the years, the continually dynamic and elastic practice structure has allowed it to adapt in an ever-changing health care environment, which includes involving the astute health care consumer in her care while maintaining the original standards and philosophies of the birth center model and the physician's office. Replication of this collaborative birth center model is one possible solution to address needed reform in maternity care and the growing problems, such as access to care, demand for limited interventions in pregnancy and birth, poor maternity outcomes, the impending maternity care workforce crisis, and the need for more options for care of vulnerable populations. To assist in possible replication, this article describes the history of the practice, the practice structure, and the collaborative practice model, and provides statistics showing evidence of successes.

## HISTORY OF THE COLLABORATIVE PRACTICE

The history of the Reading Birth and Women's Center began with its opening in 1987. At that time, the current physician was approached by a midwife who had a successful private practice in the community to see if he would be interested in being a collaborating obstetrician. Unfamiliar with midwives, yet recalling the advice of his residency director who strongly recommended that he work with midwives if given the opportunity, he accepted the offer. The birth center at the heart of this collaborative practice model is located in eastern Pennsylvania. Within the center, full gynecologic, family planning, and prenatal care is provided to a very diverse female population. Births are attended in the local hospital, the birth center, and the home. The original birth center collaborative model was initiated by Susan Stapleton, the founding midwife who worked for many years, sometimes in a hostile environment, to build relationships with local obstetricians and hospitals. By demonstrating independent midwifery care with impressive statistics, trust developed in the quality of her care and the birth center concept, allowing true collaboration to emerge. Her tireless efforts included working with the American Association of Birth Centers (AABC) to create policies, standards for accreditation, and clear collaborative guidelines for the benefit of all future midwives and birth centers. This strong foundation was essential as she transitioned out of her directorship role in 2007 and sold the birth center to her long-time collaborating obstetrician.

An obstetrician-owned birth center is a unique practice model. According to the AABC, fewer than 5% of accredited birth centers are owned by obstetricians; most birth centers are owned by midwives (Kate Bauer, personal communication, 2010). Currently, one physician and four midwives provide obstetric and gynecologic care in this collaborative practice. Both the medical and midwifery models of care are practiced and appreciated. The physician enjoys a full and challenging practice as the sole physician and owner of his own practice and the freestanding birth center. The midwives continue to provide full-scope, independent midwifery care at the birth center and to attend births in the hospital, the birth center, and the home.

## PRACTICE STRUCTURE

As the physician assumed ownership of the birth center, the practice structure was modified. The birth center has transitioned from two certified nurse midwives and one part-time nurse practitioner at the birthing center to four certified nurse midwives and two practice sites-the birth center and the OB/GYN office. Two of the full-time certified nurse midwives share the role of director, which has been divided into Administrative Director, who manages both offices and coordinates financial and business issues, and Clinical Director, who overseas clinical issues. The third full-time midwife coordinates staff in-services, coordinates the provider's schedules, and helps maintain the birth center's "Baby-Friendly" designation. All report to the collaborating obstetrician and owner of the practice. The midwives take first call, with the physician being readily available and on call at all times.

Only the midwives rotate regularly between the two offices and provide gynecologic and obstetric care in both locations. The birth center is staffed by a midwife and a registered nurse on call 24 hours a day, 7 days a week, whereas many others support the entire practice (**Table 1**).

Communication is the key to collaborative relationships, and although time-consuming, it is crucial for success. In this practice, regular communication includes weekly staff meetings involving both offices and scheduled regular communication between the providers. Clinical communication includes weekly chart review of new obstetric clients, monthly chart review of women with specific issues of concern, and quarterly chart review of births with unexpected outcomes or increased interventions during birth. Emergency drills for birth are performed regularly with clinical birth center staff, and once a year with local ambulance and hospital staff.

Supplementary to the clinical meetings, administrative meetings occur twice yearly, which include the owner, both directors, and a community member, who is a client of the practice, to review policies and procedures, budget, and long-term planning.

In addition to scheduled chart reviews, communication about clients and clinical issues occurs via in-person discussions, phone consultations, collaborative worksheets, and progress note–sharing via fax to and from the physician, and a secure Web-based information storage program that is password-protected and accessible by all providers in the practice. In the near future, the practice will be converting from traditional charting to an electronic medical record system.

The weekly staff meetings include nursing, clerical, medical, and midwifery staff. Staff meetings have an agenda and a roundtable discussion for all to openly share concerns and triumphs. The joint meetings have assisted in a smoother transition and merging of the practices. Because collaboration occurs among all staff, they feel valued and are willing to approach any of the providers to discuss issues or

**Table 1**
**Staffing for entire practice**

| Staff | FTE | Duties |
|---|---|---|
| Registered Nurse (RN) | 2.75 Full Time Equivalent (FTE) | Contraceptive management office visits, telephone triage, home visits, 1 wk postpartum visits, birth assistant, ordering of supplies, sterilizing equipment, venipuncture, and quality assurance |
| Medical technicians | 3.25 FTE | Office support, assisting in office visits, processing laboratory specimens, maintaining rooms and equipment, assist providers as needed |
| Clerical staff | 7 FTE | Scheduling all appointments, answering phone calls, clerical work, and smooth running of office |
| Lactation consultant (per diem) | 0.25 FTE | Available for all OB clients through 6 wks postpartum as needed, then as needed (PRN), provides staff in-services |
| Certified Nurse Midwife (CNM) | 4.0 FTE | Full scope OB/GYN care, first call for practice, limited third trimester ultrasound, all out of hospital care, primary providers for all birth |
| Obstetrician (OB) | 1.0 FTE | Full scope OB/GYN care in OB office only, all routine ultrasound and procedures in-office, surgeries, second call, all low transverse cesarean section and instrument-assisted births, and normal birth only if woman chooses OB as provider |

concerns as respected team members. All bring their areas of expertise to the table to contribute to the success of the whole.

With all of the staff involved, scheduling becomes very important; if the schedule does not work for everyone, nothing works. Midwifery care is time-intensive, and includes "labor sitting." The midwifery model of care requires longer office visits than are customary for an obstetrician. A commitment to out-of-hospital birth and birth at multiple locations also requires time. In this practice, the midwife on call is not scheduled in the office. She is then available to perform hospital rounds, address any problems that may arise, and attend laboring women. The midwife takes first call, and the obstetrician is always available by phone and ready to be present if needed. Time off is a valued commodity and top priority. All providers need to be flexible and committed to making the practice work. The practice is fortunate that all of the providers have the same basic philosophies regarding maternity care. Providing mutual support and backup and mutual respect for personal boundaries is important. Balance is essential.

A guiding principle for the practice has always been to provide high-quality care to all women. The birth center cares for a significant Mennonite population that is drawn to the midwifery model. Most of these women desire minimal intervention during childbirth and cost-effective care, while ensuring safe maternity care, a value set that the practice strives to embrace.

The birth center has always accepted women with Medicaid funding. Approximately 50% of the practice is Medicaid, 20% is self-pay, and the remainder is private insurance. The practice also participates in a grant program to provide income-based family planning services to women who financially qualify.

## PRINCIPLES FOR SUCCESS

A successful collaboration among the OB/GYN, midwife, and mother must embrace both the midwifery model and the medical model as equally valid and important, for they are complementary. In Pennsylvania, a certified nurse-midwife must have a collaborative agreement signed and filed with the Board of Medicine (49 Pa Code §18.1, 18.2, 18.5. Licensure and Regulation of Midwife Activities) to practice and obtain prescriptive authority.

A definition of collaboration that best describes the collaborative practice model followed in this practice is:

> *Collaboration is significantly more complex than simply working in close proximity to one another. It implies a bond, a joining together, a union and a degree of caring about one another and the relationship. A collaborative relationship is not merely the sum of its inputs. The collaborative relationship is more importantly a synergistic alliance that maximizes the contributions of each participant, resulting in an action that is greater than the sum of individual works.*[15]

A successful collaborative arrangement requires the acceptance of some basic principles. The significant characteristics of a collaborative practice described by Stapleton[16] include

- Mutual respect
- Acknowledgment of different but equally important models of care
- Joint development of and adherence to practice guidelines
- Understanding of the midwives' scope of care to avoid "taking over" or placing them in a situation beyond their expertise
- Effective and regular communication

Mutual respect allows a trust relationship to evolve and flourish. Collaboration excludes competition and eliminates negative stereotypes. Just as the midwife-mother relationship takes time to build, so does the midwife-physician relationship.

The second principle acknowledges and welcomes differences. The midwifery model of care embraces a partnership between provider and client, in which mutual vigilance and attention to detail are used to support a belief in the normalcy of the birth process. The physical structure of a free-standing birth center is welcoming to the woman and her family, and embodies and reinforces the midwifery model in all aspects of care. However, the medical model tends to be more task-oriented, focusing on managing problems and providing a foundation for intervention when required. The engaged woman requires thorough explanation of interventions that may be suggested, in a way that considers her value set. Understanding these differences and validating their separate-yet-equal importance is essential.

The third principle is that the physician and midwife together develop and agree to practice guidelines, which are always followed. These practice guidelines are referred to and useful when providers are debating appropriateness of care and management of cases, thus keeping them true to the center's philosophy. The guidelines are also dynamic and changing as research evolves and as each member contributes to them. They are reviewed yearly and updated as needed to reflect current practice.

Evidence-based practice is valued. Without equivocation, the physician in this practice feels that the collaborative relationships he and the midwives have developed are the most positive step in his career development as an obstetrician. The midwives he has worked with have insisted on evidence-based medicine before it was the buzz-word of the 21st century. For example, early in his role as a collaborating physician, the midwives were able to show that the incidence rates of third- and fourth-degree lacerations in their practice were a fraction of the rates in the hospital obstetric department because the midwives did not perform routine episiotomies. Many more examples have contributed to a primary cesarean rate of 9.5% and a successful vaginal birth after cesarean rate of 73% (**Table 2**).

**Table 2**
**Birth center statistics: a 3-year summary (2008–2010)**

| | |
|---|---|
| Total births (n) | 921–29 planned LTCS = 892 |
| Births by CNMs | 775 (87%) |
| Spontaneous vaginal delivery | 788 (88%) |
| Unplanned primary LTCS | 85 (9.5%) |
| Assisted vaginal deliveries | 19 (2%) |
| Successful vaginal birth after cesarean section | 43 (73%) |
| Preterm labor and delivery | 19 (2%) |
| Induction of labor | 177 (19.7%) |
| Augmentation of labor | 133 (14.8%) |
| Epidural rate | 269 (29%) |
| Third-/fourth-degree laceration | 11 (1%) |
| Intrapartum referral rate from out of hospital | 35 (8%) |
| Antepartum referral rate (collaboration with OB); includes phone consult and co-management | 202 (22%) |
| Annual well-woman examinations (all providers) | >3000 |

*Abbreviation:* LTCS, low transverse cesarean section.

In Pennsylvania, certified nurse-midwives are autonomous providers with prescriptive authority and access to laboratories and hospitals. As long as collaborative partners work within their licensure, scope of practice, and collaborative guidelines, each is protected from vicarious liability. These guidelines must be carefully constructed, reviewed, and updated regularly by all parties involved, while remaining evidence-based.

The fourth principle is that the physician understands the scope of midwifery practice. The physician and midwives are available to each other for ongoing consultation and collaboration. The midwives understand their scope and practice within it at all times. The physician is readily available when needed and also understands a midwife's scope of practice and each midwife's level of expertise. Commitment from the OB/GYN is needed because the choice to collaborate with midwives can be criticized.

Not everyone embraces the midwifery philosophy or understands the value of independent midwifery care or the significant difference between collaboration and supervision. Supervision is oversight and direction of care. Collaboration is a relationship between autonomous participants, which requires time and effort to develop. Acts of supervision, which include cosigning of patient charts, repeating examinations, and other supervisory behavior, can be confusing to the mother, frustrating to the practicing midwife, and time-consuming for the physician, and could extend the physician's liability.[17–19] Supervisory behavior should be discouraged at all times. The support of the collaborating physician both clinically and politically prevents placing the midwives in a position of jeopardy. The role of the collaborating physician is fluid and dynamic. The obstetrician's participation constantly changes as the clinical scenario unfolds, ranging from a simple phone call consultation to a request for immediate assistance.

The fifth principle is for the midwife to engage in effective regular communication regarding anticipation of a potential problem. The midwives are taught the art of anticipation and are committed to never surprising the obstetrician with a previously known and now immediate crisis. It is always best for the midwife to voice concerns about a potential situation rather than to call the obstetrician for the first time in the midst of a crisis. At the same time, the obstetrician must be readily available and open to respond to the midwife's need for consultation.

All partners in the collaboration must embrace these principles and have respect for and trust in each other. Mutual interdependence is the key to success. The center's insurance carrier has confirmed that liability exposure in the practice structure is actually decreased, largely because of the collaborative relationship among the physician and midwives.[10] The decrease in liability is also attributed to the trust-based relationship between midwife and mother that is extended to the collaborating physician through their work together.[17,18]

Besides providing evidence-based maternity care, another positive aspect to collaborative care is the benefit of empowering the client with partnership in the decision-making process about her care. Through empowerment, trust develops between the care provider and the client, and the client demonstrates greater compliance with the care plan.

## WORKING TOGETHER FOR QUALITY OUTCOMES

The outcomes of this collaborative practice are strong. The statistics are averaged and include data over a 3-year period from January 2008 through December 2010 for the entire practice. Some pertinent rates include: 921 total births, 87% of which were attended by midwives, and a vaginal birth rate of 88% (see **Table 2**).

In 2010, the antepartum referral rate, also known as the collaborative rate, was 22.6%. Because of regular communication between providers, when a complication emerges, often the woman does not need to leave the primary care of the midwives. When a referral is made to the collaborating physician, the patient stays within the practice for joint management of care with the midwives and obstetrician. The most common antepartum cases, which were referred to the physician and jointly managed in 2010, included gestational diabetes, hypertensive disorders, nonreassuring fetal testing, postdate inductions, hypothyroidism, multiple gestation, and other conditions, such as anencephaly, seizure disorder, and cholestasis of pregnancy. The providers have also seen more than 3000 women who presented for annual gynecologic examinations (see **Table 2**).

A discussion of a collaborative practice would not be comprehensive without including data on finances. Before the final merging of the birth center and OB/GYN practices, the physician charged a consultant fee for services rendered, and the additional revenue was added to the bottom line of the physician's practice. The birth center clients who were in need of gynecologic surgical care were referred to the physician practice. Through the years this created a stable surgical population, although the additional revenue is difficult to quantify.

When the two practices merged in 2007, the payroll needed to be expanded. Two additional midwives were hired along with some additional office staff, which initially put a strain on cash flow. Eventually, the practice saw greater than 5% increase in revenues between 2009 and 2010, which translated into an increased profit of roughly 3%. This increase occurred despite a difficult economy and its accompanying constraints.

## UNEXPECTED BENEFITS

The practice has worked diligently toward the goal of providing a changing paradigm of maternity care that is more integrative and collaborative while allowing pregnant women the freedom to choose the type of maternity care provider and location for birth they desire. Clients benefit from this collaborative practice model in which there is a seamless and complete access to care no matter what their financial status, health needs, or choice of birth provider or location.

Some positive outcomes cannot be measured by statistics. The midwives' continuing presence on the maternity units of the local hospital reinforces the years of groundwork laid by midwives such as the birth center's founder. Many of the original efforts made by pioneering midwives have had a continued positive impact on the culture at the local hospital. Thirty years ago, midwives did not have hospital privileges, and some bedside nurses blocked midwives' attempt to remain at the bedside with the client. Conversely, the hospital nurses have recently formed a committee on natural childbirth focusing on reeducation and sensitivity training for all staff on the labor floor to provide better care for clients who choose less intervention. The hospital where the members of this practice have privileges also now has its own midwifery practice that works closely with the OB/GYN residency program.

The use of principles from the collaborative model extends beyond the relationship of the four midwives and physician to interdisciplinary relationships formed in the hospital setting, including pediatricians, lactation consultants, and social workers. Multidisciplinary breastfeeding initiatives have encouraged 24-hour rooming in and more on-staff lactation consultants. Clients now have the option of early discharge when appropriate to their care needs.

Now when a need exists for client transfer from an out-of-hospital setting to the hospital, there is an expedient flow of information and a willingness of hospital nursing staff and resident physicians to offer assistance as needed. The culture has changed and now participation is seen as an opportunity to experience a unique model of care. The midwives have the benefit of hospital credentials with admitting privileges, allowing a seamless transition for the client to the hospital when additional intervention is indicated.

## EDUCATIONAL OPPORTUNITIES

The birth center serves as a clinical site for those wanting to learn about the midwifery model of care, including medical residents, nursing students, midwifery students, childbirth educators, and doulas. Every effort is made to offer educational opportunities and encourage a learning environment while keeping the personal, home-like environment of the birth center intact. When asked permission first, clients are generally very gracious about allowing observation or participation of students. Requesting permission is part of the midwifery model in which a relationship is established with the woman based on mutual respect and trust. Recently, an OB/GYN intern contacted the practice wishing to observe an out-of-hospital birth. She felt this was an important part of her clinical education and would help to keep her grounded in the original reason she went to medical school. Midwifery students and medical residents, including family practice residents, are welcomed to observe and potentially participate in the practice's monthly chart reviews and biannual transfer reviews (cases that were for out-of-hospital birth but were transferred for a hospital birth for a specific reason). The practice of reviewing cases through chart review allows observers to see the process of collaboration unfold, because all participants' comments are valued and viewed as equally important. These meetings involve discussions of clinical situations and a critical review of care that is currently being provided, and discussions regarding past cases, current practice guidelines, and opportunities for improvement.

## REPLICATION OF THE MODEL

This model can be reproduced in many ways, but the authors believe some basic elements are essential. Along with the principles of collaboration, the most crucial aspect of replication is communication. Input from all people in the practice is necessary. This communication must be established in an organized manner and must occur with regularity to be productive. Providing client-focused care is at the core of success. Clients are consumers. They come to a midwifery practice with many expectations. Clients expect honesty and transparency, not patronization. The respect the staff show each other extends to their clients. When respect is the driving force behind care provided, people notice, they come back, and they bring their friends and neighbors. This practice does very little advertising, yet it continues to grow by word of mouth. Women share in the responsibility for their care. Every woman is treated as an individual with unique needs. Consent is not informed; instead, decision making is shared and is based on evidence. If a disagreement in the plan of care arises, it is discussed until the providers and the woman come to a consensus while keeping both the evidence and the woman's needs as the driving forces behind the decision. It is important to listen to the needs of the woman. Listening to the woman dictates the plan of care.

Finally, to establish an integrated, collaborative practice, it needs to have a financial base with some depth. The payroll must be met and sometimes cash flow is sporadic and undependable in a medical practice. Having a working budget and spending plan is very important.

## SUMMARY

The physician was wise to follow his residency instructor's advice to take advantage of an opportunity to work with midwives if possible. The physician's residency instructor had his training in England, and he predicted that the midwifery model would someday be the most efficient way to use an obstetrician's training in obstetric complications by placing uncomplicated obstetric care into the hands of those who were best suited to deliver that care. Currently, all of the providers enjoy what they consider a perfect practice. The midwives have had a large increase in the volume of obstetric clients while the physician remains available for obstetric issues. The midwives are able to concentrate on education and forming partnerships with the obstetric and gynecologic clients, and the physician is able to focus on developing a busy gynecologic surgical practice. The arrangement has resulted in a flourishing practice in midwifery care, safe and evidence-based obstetric care, and a blossoming gynecologic surgical practice, which has increased more than 100% over the past 3 years. This collaborative practice has allowed each provider to excel in their area of expertise while pursuing the common goal of high-quality, cost-effective maternity and gynecologic care and a safe labor and birth, individualized for each woman.

## ACKNOWLEDGMENTS

With special acknowledgments to Susan R. Stapleton, DNP, CNM, FACNM, for her pioneering birth center and collaborating practice foundations; to Rebecca K. Jones, MD, for her guidance and topic development toward this manuscript; and to Deborah Weitkamp, RN, BSN, for her editorial contributions.

## REFERENCES

1. Merriam Webster's Online Dictionary. Available at: http://www.merriam-webster.com/dictionary/collaborate. Accessed January 13, 2011.
2. Hess RG. From bedside to boardroom: nursing shared governance. Online J Issues Nurs 2004;9(1):2.
3. Haller G, Garnerin P, Morales MA, et al. Effect of crew resource management training in a multidisciplinary obstetrical setting. Int J Qual Health Care 2008; 20(4):254–63.
4. Skinner J, Foureur M. Consultation, referral, and collaboration between midwives and obstetricians: lessons from New Zealand. J Midwifery Womens Health 2010; 55(1):28–37.
5. O'Brien B, Harvey S, Sommerfeldt S, et al. Comparison of costs and associated outcomes between women choosing newly integrated autonomous midwifery care and matched controls: a pilot study. J Obstet Gynaecol Can 2010;32(7): 650–6.
6. Institute of Medicine. Prenatal care: reaching mothers, reaching infants. Washington, DC: National Academy Press; 1988.
7. Institute of Medicine. For the public's health: the role of measurement in action and accountability. Institute of Medicine of the National Academies. Available at: http://iom.edu/Reports/2010/For-the-Publics-Health-The-Role-of-Measurement-in-Action-and-Accountability/Report-Brief.aspx. Accessed January 26, 2011.
8. MacDorman MF, Mathews TJ. Recent trends in infant mortality in the United States. NCHS data brief, no. 9. Hyattsville (MD): National Center for Health Statistics; 2008.

9. Sakala C, Corry M. Evidence-based maternity care: what it is and what it can achieve. New York: Milbank Memorial Fund; 2008.
10. Jackson D, Lang JM, Swartz WH, et al. Outcomes, safety, and resource utilization in a collaborative care birth center program compared with traditional physician-based perinatal care. Am J Public Health 2003;93(6):999–1006.
11. Carter MC, Corry M, Delbanco S, et al. 2020 vision for a high-quality, high-value maternity care system. Womens Health Issues 2010;20(Suppl 1):S7–17.
12. World Health Organization. The millennium development goals report. New York: United Nations; 2010.
13. Fox S. The engaged e-patient population. The Pew Internnet. Available at: http://www.pewinternet.org/Reports/2008/The-Engaged-Epatient-Population/The-Engaged-E-patient-Population.aspxn. Accessed January 6, 2012.
14. Epstien A. The business of being born [DVD]. New York: Red Envelope Entertainment and New Line Home Entertainment; 2008.
15. Evans J. The role of the nurse manager in creating an environment of collaborative practice. Holist Nurs Pract 1994;8(3):22–31.
16. Stapleton SR. Team-building: making collaborative practice work. J Nurse Midwifery 1998;43(1):12–8.
17. Jenkins S. The myth of vicarious liability. J Nurse Midwifery 1994;39(2):98–106.
18. Woods JR, Rozovsky FA. What do I say? Communicating intended or unanticipated outcomes in obstetrics. San Francisco (CA): John Wiley & Sons; 2003.
19. King T, Summers L. Is collaborative practice a malpractice risk? Myth versus reality. J Midwifery Womens Health 2005;5(6):451–2.

# Midwives and Obstetrician-Gynecologists Collaborating for Native American Women's Health

Joseph A. (Tony) Ogburn, MD[a,*], Eve Espey, MD, MPH[a], Marilyn Pierce-Bulger, CNM, FNP, MN[b], Alan Waxman, MD, MPH[a], Lisa Allee, CNM[c], William H.J. Haffner, MD[d], Jean Howe, MD, MPH[c]

**KEYWORDS**

• Certified nurse-midwives • Obstetrician-gynecologists • Native American women

**KEY POINTS**

- Collaborative care between CNMs and Obstetrician-gynecologists physicians in the Indian Health Service has contributed to improved health outcomes for mothers and infants.
- Collaborative care is a cost effective approach that optimizes the use of resources in low resource settings.
- Collaborative care enables providers to practice at the top of their skill level and provides flexibility in the expansion of practice activities.
- An environment of mutual respect and open communication is critical to the success of collaborative practice.

## INTRODUCTION

Certified Nurse-Midwives (CNMs) and Obstetrician-gynecologists (OBGs) have a long and successful history of collaboration in serving Native American women. Their roles are complementary: CNMs provide holistic, patient-centered care and OBGs provide specialty consultative services for complicated medical problems and/or surgical intervention. CNMs have a long history of practice within the Indian Health Service (IHS) and Tribal systems of care. Native American women are more likely than any other ethnic group in the United States to be attended at child birth by CNMs, providers who are

Source: University of New Mexico. Disclosures: None. Funding: None.
[a] Department of Obstetrics and Gynecology, MSC 10 5580, University of New Mexico, Albuquerque, NM 87131, USA; [b] Alaska Native Medical Center/Southcentral Foundation, 4320 Diplomacy Drive, Anchorage, AK 95008, USA; [c] Northern Navajo Medical Center, PO Box 160, Highway 491 N, Shiprock, NM 87420; [d] Department of Obstetrics and Gynecology, Uniformed Services University of the Health Sciences, 4301 Jones Bridge Road, Bethesda, MD 20814, USA
* Corresponding author.
*E-mail address:* jogburn@salud.unm.edu

Obstet Gynecol Clin N Am 39 (2012) 359–366
http://dx.doi.org/10.1016/j.ogc.2012.05.004
0889-8545/12/$ – see front matter 

educated in the 2 disciplines of nursing and midwifery.[1] CNMs are educated to recognize deviations from normal, consult or refer when indicated, and promote the health and well-being of women, mothers, and infants. The style of practice of CNMs aligns well with the Native American values in which, historically, the indigenous women were assisted by female relatives and tribal midwives during child birth. Birth is viewed as a normal event within the context of family and community life. The nurse-midwifery role has long been recognized within the IHS system as a valued service that is medically and culturally appropriate. The combination of nurse-midwifery care for normal labor and comanagement for complicated problems has resulted in outstanding comprehensive maternity care for Native American women.

This article summarizes the history of collaborative care in the IHS, describes several examples of current successful collaborative practices, and discusses keys to successful collaborative practice in the IHS setting that may apply to other practice settings.

## HISTORY OF COLLABORATIVE MATERNITY CARE IN THE IHS

From the late 1960s, many IHS facilities employed CNMs to provide maternity care. Two IHS hospitals on the Navajo reservation: the Fort Defiance Indian Hospital in northeastern Arizona and the Shiprock Indian Hospital in northwestern New Mexico, provided collaborative midwife-physician care. These hospitals served as formal training sites for the midwifery educational programs of the Johns Hopkins University and the University of Utah. In western Alaska, IHS general practice physicians informally collaborated with the tribal doctor/healer Rita Blumenstein. After the successful experience with Blumenstein, the IHS integrated a CNM into their provider groups at Bethel, Alaska and at the Alaska Native Medical Center (ANMC) in the early 1970s. Within a decade, CNMs were providing a majority of obstetric care at many IHS facilities. The role of the CNM varied with the size, staffing, and needs of the service unit. For example, by the mid-1970s the CNMs at Fort Defiance were offering prenatal, intrapartum, and postpartum care whereas the single CNM at nearby Gallup Indian Medical Center (GIMC) limited her practice to prenatal and well-woman care. The lone CNM at the ANMC in Anchorage attended to labor and delivery during the day shift whereas the facility's 4 OBGs rotated the night call.

In the Alaska area, changes in maternity care were motivated by the recognition that American Indian and Alaska Natives had a disproportionate share of high-risk pregnant women and that maternal and infant mortality rates were more than twice as high than those of the general US population. Recognizing this problem, Dr Beryl Blue Spruce, 1 of only 4 full-blooded American Indian physicians at the time, proposed the establishment of an Indian Health Committee by the American College of Obstetricians and Gynecologists (ACOG). In 1970, the Ad Hoc Committee on American Indian Affairs was formed under the chairmanship of Edward Zimmerman, MD, of the University of New Mexico. At the Committee's inception, ACOG president Dr J. Robert Willson recommended the inclusion of Lucille Woodville, president of the American College of Nurse Midwives (ACNM) as a liaison member.

Among the committee's first activities in 1973 to 1974 was the evaluation of the high infant mortality rate among American Indians and Alaska Natives through a series of visits to the sites. It was noted that maternity care at many facilities was provided by General Medical Officers (GMOs), who often had little obstetric training beyond medical school. The committee recommended that ACOG and IHS together develop a structured postgraduate course for the GMOs and general clinical nurses. The planning committee for the postgraduate course included OBGs, CNMs, and pediatricians from the IHS and from academic referral centers familiar with the high-risk population of the IHS. The curriculum was developed in the late 1970s and the first course was conducted in 1980. The course is still offered every 1 to 2 years. During this time, many IHS service units recognized the benefits of CNMs and began employing them instead of GMOs to provide maternity care.

In the mid-1970s the Indian Health Service Manual was published with a chapter devoted to maternal and child health. This chapter was developed by the senior consultants in obstetrics, nurse-midwifery, and pediatrics and provided guidelines for maternity care. It required that programs have a formal relationship with a local or regional OBG as well as a regional high-risk referral center. Even in remote areas, the IHS model of collaborative practice between CNMs and OBGs was the standard of care.

By 1997, CNMs and OBGs worked together throughout the IHS. Larger regional medical centers, such as the Phoenix Indian Medical Center (PIMC) (7 OBGs and 8 CNMs), and GIMC (6 OBGs and 6 CNMs), had birth volumes of more than 900 per year. These facilities employed CNMs to cover all routine prenatal and inpatient maternity care. OBGs provided consultation for complicated obstetric patients and specialty gynecology services. At smaller facilities such as Santa Fe Indian Hospital with fewer than 300 births per year, the 3 CNMs and 2 OBGs shared the workload.

The scope of practice and nature of collaboration varied as well. At PIMC, low-risk women were admitted to the CNM service and high-risk patients to an OBG service. Low-risk patients who developed complications were transferred to the OBG service. By contrast, at GIMC and Chinle Comprehensive Health Care Facility (CCHCF), CNMs managed patients in routine laboring but co-managed patients with more complications with the OBG. The CNMs managed labor and attended the birth, whereas the OBG managed the complicating condition.

## *Current Collaborative Practice*

The majority of IHS and Tribal sites that provide maternity care now employ midwives, practicing collaboratively with OBGs or Family Medicine physicians depending on the site's needs and resources (**Table 1**). Clinical outcomes such as cesarean delivery and VBAC rates are much lower than the national averages (**Table 2**). Reasons for these positive outcomes are complex, but are significantly influenced by the collaborative midwifery-obstetric model.

CNMs serve in clinical practice and leadership positions within and across departments as clinical preceptors for medical students, residents, nurse practitioner, and nurse-midwifery students. They are involved in quality assurance and clinical decision-making activities. Depending on the needs of a site and the interests of the CNMs, they may expand their scope of practice to include colposcopy, ultrasonography, forensic examinations of sexual assault, obstetric vacuum extraction, and first assisting at cesarean deliveries. These expanded roles have received the support of IHS and the ACNM. The mechanism for attainment of new skills is described within the ACNM Standards for the Practice of Midwifery.[2]

IHS and tribal nurse-midwives have been responsible for the development of many model programs for women and infants in their respective communities. One example is the Alaska Southcentral Foundation's Nutaqsiivik Program, a home visitation pilot project developed in 1994 for American Indian/Alaska Native pregnant women and their infants in the Anchorage area.[3] This project on quality improvement process demonstrating a 50% reduction in postneonatal infant mortality rate developed into an important continuing Southcentral Foundation program.

Another successful program is the expansion of the Centering Model of group prenatal care. Centering group prenatal care[4] was created by nurse-midwives and

**Table 1**
**Overview of IHS and tribal sites 2009**

| | Ada | ANMC | Chinle | Claremore | FDIH | GIMC | PIMC | Pine Ridge | SF | Shiprock | Tahlequah | Tuba |
|---|---|---|---|---|---|---|---|---|---|---|---|---|
| OBG FTE | 3 | 8.5 | 5 | 3 | 4 | 7 | 8 | 1 | 1 | 5 | 6 | 5 |
| OBG vacancy | 0 | 3.5 | 1 | 2 | 1 | 0 | 1 | 1 | 0 | 1 | 1 | 0 |
| CNM FTE | 4 | 9 | 7 | 5 | 6 | 6 | 8 | 7 | 3 | 5 | 7 | 7 |
| CNM vacancy | 0 | 0 | 3 | 2 | 0 | 1 | 0 | 3 | 0 | 1 | 0 | 0 |

*Abbreviations:* FDIH, Fort Defiance Indian Hospital; FTE, Full time equivalents; GIMC, Gallup Indian Medical Center; PIMC, Phoenix Indian Medical Center; SF, Sante fe.
*From* Jean Howe, IHS Chief Clinical Consultant for Ob/Gyn; with permission.

**Table 2**
**Navajo area birth statistics (2009)**

| | Chinle | FDIH | Gallup | Shiprock | Tuba City | Total |
|---|---|---|---|---|---|---|
| Births | 541 | 459 | 664 | 763 | 519 | 2946 |
| Vaginal | 457 | 383 | 570 | 586 | 420 | 2416 |
| 1° C/S | 52 (9.6%) | 47 (10.2%) | 55 (8.4%) | 83 (10.9%) | 53 (10.2%) | 290 (9.8%) |
| R C/S | 32 (5.9%) | 29 (6.3%) | 39 (5.9%) | 94 (12.3%) | 46 (8.7%) | 240 (8.1%) |
| Total C/S | 84 | 76 | 94 | 177 | 99 | 530 |
| C/S Rate | 15.5% | 16.5% | 14.2% | 23.2% | 19.1% | 18.0% |
| VBAC | 20 | 20 | 36 | 21 | 16 | 113 |
| VBAC % | 3.7% | 4.4% | 5.4% | 2.8% | 3.1% | 3.8% |
| VBAC Success % | 71.4% | 90.9% | 87.8% | 87.5% | 80% | — |

*Abbreviation:* C/S, cesarean section.
*From* Jean Howe–IHS Chief Clinical Consultant for Ob/Gyn; with permission.

is actively supported within the IHS. Group care reduces preterm births in women-compared with standard care.[5] This model promotes self-care, includes an educational component, and becomes a support group and social connection for women. Many IHS and tribal CNMs and OBGs have participated in training supported by the IHS and now include group care as an option for patients. Anecdotal evidence from ANMC nursing staff indicates that women receiving such care are more knowledgeable and prepared for the birthing experience. This care model also fits well with the historical indigenous model of pregnancy and birth as a community event.

### *Current Collaborative Models*

One of the keys to the success of maternity care in IHS and tribal facilities is the flexibility afforded by collaborative practice. Specific examples of collaborative models are given below.

One of the founding midwives of the CCHCF, Ursula Knoki-Wilson, is the daughter of a traditional midwife who helped establish midwifery services at Chinle and provided historical and cultural context for the service. At CCHCF, midwifery was an integral part of maternity care from its inception. Midwives value the obstetricians for their skills in managing complications and obstetricians value the skills of CNMs in supporting and enhancing the normal healthy processes of pregnancy, birth, and breastfeeding. All pregnant women receive care from a CNM with consultation with an OBG as indicated. Labor and birth units are staffed by CNMs at all times, and even in high-risk settings, the CNM attends birth in collaboration with the OBG. Patients receive midwifery care, support, and encouragement for their labor and childbirth regardless of complications. Midwives attend more than 95% of the vaginal deliveries at Chinle.

ANMC serves as the level II referral facility for the statewide tribally operated hospitals and clinics. Approximately, half of the clients are from communities beyond Anchorage, and many have increased health risks. CNMs provide full scope services to all prenatal patients and consult with or refer to an OBG or perinatologist as indicated. Locally developed evidence-based practice guidelines provide a framework for clinical management. This model provides optimal care to patients and enables the OBGs to focus on specialty care in high-risk obstetrics and specialty gynecology.

The roles of CNM have recently expanded to include the provision of services within the Primary Care Clinic system, using a medical home model. Over the past year, prenatal and nonspecialty women's health care have been provided within the medical home. CNMs serve as a women's health resource for other members of the medical home team, and OBGs are available for consultation for more complicated problems. Feedback about this new collaboration from primary-care providers and patients has been positive.

#### *Challenges of the collaborative model of care*

There are certainly challenges to be resolved in order for a collaborative model to be successful. The IHS has always had to provide care with scarce resources. Depending on the needs of an individual site, there may be conflicts about providing routine care with CNMs versus staffing for the infrequent adverse event that requires the specialty services of an OBG and an anesthesia provider.

On occasion, the need for a provider with a broader clinical practice, for example, a family medicine physician, has led to the demise of a midwifery position. There have also been conflicts with the sharing of delivery volume with family medicine physicians.

OBGs and CNMs may experience tensions related to their specific roles because there is considerable overlap with a collaborative model of care. As the acuity level of care has increased in obstetrics, midwives have responded by expanding their expertise. OBGs who have not developed an understanding of the benefits of the midwifery role, a level of trust, and/or effective communication with his/her CNM colleague may find their own professional role identity in transition, which can create significant discomfort. An experienced CNM in Alaska observed that an OBG who trained with or worked previously with CNMs is more likely to engage in a satisfying, mutually rewarding collaborative practice with midwives and physicians.

***Keys to successful collaboration: lessons learned from IHS and tribal settings***

There are several reasons that explain the success of CNM-OBG collaborative practice model in IHS and Tribal facilities. The single-payer system of care that characterizes these facilities is a model in which collaborative practice is cost-effective and efficient. Providers are salaried and have no financial incentives for performing procedures. In obstetrics, for example, OBGs do not have economic incentives to perform low-risk vaginal deliveries and may focus on complicated medical problems and/or operative deliveries. Program managers can design systems in which providers' skills are best utilized. CNMs provide care for low-risk patients whereas OBGs, as specialists, provide high-risk Obstetric care and specialty gynecology. Providers in IHS and Tribal facilities are covered by the Federal Tort Claims Act, which enables providers to practice evidence-based care with less emphasis on defensive medicine.

Another reason for success is the position of a director of midwifery who provides supervision and direction to the CNM group. The IHS model includes this role at most facilities and is usually an equal to the director of the OBGs. The role of a CNM director brings validity to the midwifery service as a discipline that is equal and complimentary to, but separate from, the obstetric discipline.

Well-delineated scope of practice guidelines are very useful to ensure both CNMs and OBGs understand the role each will have in patient care. These guidelines will vary among practices, but it must be clearly defined which patients are eligible for CNM care, when referral or consultation should be obtained, and whether a transfer of care or ongoing collaborative care will occur. Expectations must be clear and adhered to or conflict may result.

An environment of respect and open communication is essential to success. Joint activities foster the spirit of collaboration. AtGIMC, educational activities such as Journal Club, peer review such as Morbidity and Mortality Conferences, and clinical practice activities (eg, a Breastfeeding Task Force) have brought CNMs and OBGs together. CNMs and OBGs working together in all aspects of practice will develop a mutual respect for the complimentary yet different skill sets that each discipline brings to the table.

## SUMMARY

In the IHS, collaborative practice of CNMs and OBGs has become the predominant model of maternity care. This model provides Native American women with high-quality care that is in harmony with their culture, is cost effective, and results in excellent outcomes. In a system of scarce resources, the evolution of collaborative practice has enabled the IHS and tribal facilities to reduce adverse outcomes to low levels while achieving the positive outcomes of low rates of cesarean delivery and high rates of successful VBAC. The success of collaborative care in the care of Native American women is an example of how CNMs and OBGs can work together to optimize maternity care for all women.

## ACKNOWLEDGMENTS

The authors would like to thank Terry Friend, CNM and Sue Rooks, CNM for their assistance in information gathering.

## REFERENCES

1. American College of nurse-midwives quickinfo- midwives serving in Indian Country. Available at: http://www.midwife.org/siteFiles/education/Indian_Country_3.3.06.pdf. Accessed November 26, 2011.
2. American College of nurse-midwives standards for the practice of midwifery 12/4/09. Available at: http://www.midwife.org/siteFiles/descriptive/Standards_for_Practice_of_Midwifery_12_09_001.pdf. Accessed November 26, 2011.
3. Pierce-Bulger M, Nighswander T. Nutaqsiivik: an approach to reducing infant mortality. Qual Manag Health Care 2001;9(3):40–6. Centering Healthcare Institute. Available at: http://www.centeringhealthcare.org/pages/about/history.php. Accessed November 26, 2011.
4. Centering Healthcare Institute. Available at: http://www.centeringhealthcare.org/pages/about/history.php. Accessed June 25, 2012.
5. Ickovics JR, Kershaw TS, Wesdahl C, et al. Group Prenatal Care and Perinatal Outcome. Obstet Gynecol 2007;110(2 Pt 1):330–9.

# A Successful Model of Collaborative Practice in a University-Based Maternity Care Setting

May Hsieh Blanchard, MD*, Jan M. Kriebs, CNM, MSN

**KEYWORDS**

- Collaborative practice • Maternity care • Residency training • Medical education

**KEY POINT**

- Collaboration between physicians and midwives shows an integrated model of successful clinical care and medical education in an urban University hospital setting.

## BACKGROUND

For years, interdisciplinary education has been described and promoted as a means to enhance collaborative care.[1] In the last 3 decades, the inclusion of midwives as staff or faculty members in academic departments of obstetrics and gynecology has become more common. Models ranging from side-by-side practices[2] to active midwifery participation in medical education[3] have developed during this time. The literature on midwives in academic medical centers describes this role development and a progressive increase in the number of participating midwives.[4–6] Our experience at the University of Maryland Medical Center provides a 15-year example of a sustainable and successful collaborative practice involving physicians and midwives. The achievements of this collaborative model are further underscored by its ability to succeed in a high-acuity setting of a regional referral academic institution located in an urban setting, serving both vulnerable and insured populations. This article describes the evolution of an integrated model of clinical care and medical education at the University of Maryland.

## PRACTICE MODEL AND OUTCOMES

The University of Maryland Medical Center has provided obstetric and gynecologic care to the women of West Baltimore and the state of Maryland since the early

Department of Obstetrics, Gynecology and Reproductive Sciences, University of Maryland School of Medicine, 22 South Greene Street, N6E04 Baltimore, MD 21201, USA
* Corresponding author. Department of Obstetrics, Gynecology & Reproductive Sciences, University of Maryland School of Medicine, 11 South Paca Street, Suite 400, Baltimore, MD 21201.
*E-mail address:* mblanchard@fpi.umaryland.edu

Obstet Gynecol Clin N Am 39 (2012) 367–372
http://dx.doi.org/10.1016/j.ogc.2012.05.005 obgyn.theclinics.com

1800s. In recent history, the Department of Obstetrics, Gynecology and Reproductive Sciences was established in 1956, staffed by the traditional academic physician faculty model. The department serves as a high-risk referral center for the state and the region. Midwives were recruited to the faculty at the University of Maryland Medical Center in 1996 to expand the services offered by the faculty practice and increase the exposure of the residents and medical students to normal pregnancy and birth.

From the start, the midwives were identified as part of the clinical faculty, providing care in both private and clinic settings and attending births of the women in their caseload. At first, the educational role was limited to modeling midwifery care to the residents as they participated in caring for midwifery patients during labor and birth, in their separate midwife private practices. As the midwifery presence and practice evolved, the midwifery group became increasingly integrated and integral to the clinical and academic functions of the department. The midwives continue to directly provide care for women, including a private low-risk practice, specialty clinics for human immunodeficiency virus (HIV)–positive and young adolescent women (teen clinic), and women who are at increased medical risk but are seeking midwifery care. The group also works with medical students at both preclinical and clerkship levels, is active in the didactic education of residents and midwifery students, performs deliveries with residents, and supervises new residents and medical students in obstetric triage.

Several forces moved the Obstetrics and Gynecology Department toward an integrated model of service including (1) the demands of clinical care volumes and didactic education in a high-acuity setting, (2) the midwives' desire to participate more fully in teaching roles, (3) shifts in resident duty-hour requirements, and (4) willingness of both physicians and midwives to work collegially in this environment. The labor and delivery unit is staffed by 2 faculty members at all times, an obstetrician and a midwife, who seamlessly share patient care responsibilities; this is not to say that the duties are divided equally, because their scopes of practice differ. However, the obstetrician and midwife on duty have embraced an environment of mutual respect and collegiality, such that each supports the other. The midwife is the first line in triage, supervising the interns and junior residents as they evaluate and assess pregnant patients with a host of obstetric and nonobstetric conditions. The obstetrician is thus available for consultation on complications and for surgical intervention.

Midwifery faculty members were thoughtfully recruited and selected for strong clinical experience and flexibility to work in a model in which traditional midwifery management of labor may not be appropriate or possible. The midwives are adept at identifying when physician involvement is indicated. Meanwhile, if the physician is otherwise occupied in the operating room or the emergency department, or in gynecology-service care, the midwife is able to work with the resident staff to monitor the labor unit caseload and accomplish their births.

If there is a midwife private-practice patient who has risk factors suspicious for a complicated delivery, the physician is welcome to check on the progress of the labor managed by the midwife, and to serve as backup to a colleague. The physicians also enlist the aid of the midwives when there may be a challenging second stage of labor, receiving suggestions for different approaches to pushing and midwifery techniques that might aid in achieving a successful vaginal delivery.

Throughout this collaborative model of care, the midwives are integral to, and actively participate in, the education of every level of resident. This participation includes evaluating their history-taking and physical diagnosis skills, coaching them to develop clearer and more succinct presentation skills, assessing their hands-on technical skills during births, and monitoring and expanding their leadership and teaching skills, with their progressively increasing responsibility commensurate with their level of training. The dual-faculty presence allows for division of labor, resourcefully using the expertise of each, while ensuring constant and ongoing teaching, supervision, and evaluation of the residents. The result is enhanced education of residents and championing patient safety and delivery of quality care. Furthermore, the clinical education of the interns and junior residents is enhanced by having the opportunity to see normal births attended by the midwife faculty juxtaposed with complex births supervised by the attending physician. This system helps young residents to differentiate normal versus abnormal and to alternate and adapt to the changing clinical scenarios. Active involvement in births that range from natural birth in various maternal positions to complex premature deliveries enables the physician to draw on a wider set of skills and understanding in providing care to women.

## CREDENTIALING

One institutional challenge is the lack of admitting privileges for midwives, which is a hospital-wide issue for nonphysician providers. Midwives are credentialed as part of the affiliate rather than active staff. Although midwives are able to write their own prescriptions and see patients independently in the office setting, admissions of the patients of the midwifery practice still require a physician to be named. Midwifery practice patients would ideally be admitted under their own names and their own practice group, thus reflecting the responsibilities assumed and ownership taken. However, this has not proved to be an insurmountable barrier to independent care, as a result of the strongly collegial approach of the faculty. The hospital credentialing committee involved the Midwifery Director and Department Chair in discussion of appropriate clinical privileges. The final document provides both for midwifery management of near-term and term pregnancies and for midwifery attendance at any vaginal birth when the physician attending is in agreement or is engaged in another case and not immediately available to supervise the resident staff.

## INTERDISCIPLINARY EDUCATION AND TRAINING

Our practice offers many examples of ways in which interdisciplinary education strengthens patient care. Residency candidates are interviewed by members of the midwifery division. The participating midwife and physician faculty commit to interviewing candidates for the residency application season, to provide consistency and stability in the ranking and evaluation of the candidates. Midwives teach in the so-called intern boot camp (an intensive 8-hour preclinical orientation to clinical skills and surgical procedures for the incoming intern class each summer) and provide regular lectures for new interns during their first several months in residency training. The sessions provide guidance to the new physicians, in which questions about the basics of care can be asked and addressed in a safe, nonjudgmental environment. The obstetric simulation center, managed by midwifery faculty, is used for hands-on learning, from basic hand skills, to team drills, to remediation of specific resident learning deficits, and integrates multidisciplinary team training. Midwifery students who receive clinical training in the practice are equally exposed to this model of care and have the opportunity to work with medical students and residents. For example, the chief resident may review a triage plan of the midwifery student before it is presented to the faculty midwife, or an advanced midwifery student may have medical students observe a birth and talk about why they made certain choices about birth position and support techniques. The department incorporated the TeamSTEPPS program (developed by the Department of Defense in collaboration with the Agency for Healthcare Research and Quality)[7] with full involvement of the antepartum, intrapartum, and postpartum staff members. The education and training involved team leaders of obstetricians, midwives, nurses, and an anesthesiologist who took the initial training together. This team then led education sessions created specifically for this department, teaching the TeamSTEPPS concepts to their colleagues, encouraging open discussion, and successfully introducing techniques of communication and situational awareness to improve day-to-day patient care, safety consciousness, and hand-off processes. On a practical level, the attending physician and faculty midwife work together daily to ensure that regular briefings and huddles of the multiple stakeholders occur at scheduled intervals, even when the unit is busy.

Several aspects of our practice directly affect our ability to enhance patient safety. TeamSTEPPS training has improved communication. Triage timeliness and accuracy are improved. Two faculty members are always available to labor and delivery. In addition, the faculty clinicians are practiced at sharing both information and responsibilities, which allows smoother transitions in an emergency.

## OPPORTUNITIES

Because midwives work in a collaborative setting, opportunities to offer and provide midwifery care are increased. As a faculty, we support the option of vaginal birth after cesarean (VBAC). Women desiring VBAC can see the midwives for prenatal care and birth and there is always a physician immediately available to assist as indicated. Women with medical complications such as multiple sclerosis can have a midwife for their primary provider, with consultation from the maternal-fetal medicine division, as can women with obstetric issues such as a growth-restricted fetus. Perhaps the most developed example of this in our department is our midwifery clinic for HIV seropositive pregnant women. This practice has grown into a referral center for the community. The HIV pregnancy clinic population reflects the overall insurance mix of patients in the clinic setting. Many of the predominantly Medicaid-insured women have difficulty in accessing needed resources. The complex social and psychological stressors they face in addition to their medical needs challenge their ability to adhere to a plan of care.

Care is provided by members of the midwifery division under the leadership of the Midwifery Director, who has nationally recognized expertise in caring for the HIV seropositive pregnant population. Essential to the success of the clinic is the interdisciplinary team comprising the midwife, a maternal-fetal medicine physician with special interest in infectious diseases, social workers, peer counselors, and well-established adult and pediatric HIV medical practices. Reaching across disciplines and departments, the service has been able to maintain a perinatal HIV transmission rate of 1% to 2%. In women without care, national perinatal transmission rates may reach as high as 25%.[8] Baltimore City has been identified as one of the highest-risk areas, having the second-highest rate of new acquired immune deficiency syndrome cases in the country.[9]

Another example of midwifery integration into departmental activities is the Perinatal Outreach Service established in a neighboring county's health department clinic. A team comprising a maternal-fetal medicine physician, midwife, and sonographer provides weekly on-site consultative services for high-risk women. The clinic serves women whose risk profiles require more intense supervision than is locally available.

In addition, an integrated department offers increased opportunities for clinical research, whether that is a resident or fellow using an existing database such as the HIV clinic data, a midwife partnering with an obstetrician to study outcomes in diabetes and obesity, or clinical support offered to new researchers as they develop ideas.[10–20] The generalist obstetric and midwifery divisions are working to promote further collaboration in the research arena to address common clinical concerns in our population, such as substance abuse, obesity education, and depression.

## SUMMARY

Clinical competence does not necessarily mean identical choices in clinical management. Each party has to adapt to achieve a successful working relationship. Without mutual respect and trust, integrated models of care do not work. Physicians, traditionally viewed as the leaders of the health care team, must be able to share authority as well as responsibility, recognizing that other professionals have the education to provide autonomous care. Midwives need to be confident that a request for information or suggestion for medical intervention by an obstetric colleague is not a challenge to their competence. At the same time, working in education demands a commitment to maintaining knowledge of the supporting evidence for all choices, including those more commonly associated with midwifery practice than with medicine. There must be mutual trust and respect as cofaculty without suspicion, turf battles, or resistance to medically indicated intervention. Replication and implementation of the collaborative physician-midwifery model demonstrated at the University of Maryland requires a philosophic and hands-on investment on the part of both groups.

## REFERENCES

1. Baldwin DC. The role of interdisciplinary education and teamwork in primary care and health care reform. Rockville (MD): US Department of Health and Human Services PHS, Human Resources and Services Administration, Bureau of Health Professions, Office of Health Professions Analysis and Research; 1994. p. 92–1009.
2. Sedler KD, Lydon-Rochelle M, Castillo YM, et al. Nurse-midwifery service model in an academic environment. J Nurse Midwifery 1993;38(4):241–5.
3. Angelini DJ, Afriat CI, Hodgman DE, et al. Development of an academic nurse-midwifery service program. A partnership model between medicine and midwifery. J Nurse Midwifery 1996;41(3):236–42.
4. Long WN, Sharp ES. Relationships between professions: from the viewpoint of the physician and nurse-midwife in a tertiary center. J Nurse Midwifery 1982; 27(4):14–24.
5. McConaughey E, Howard E. Midwives as educators of medical students and residents: results of a national survey. J Midwifery Womens Health 2009;54(4): 268–74.
6. Platt LD, Angelini DJ, Paul RH, et al. Nurse-midwifery in a large teaching hospital. Obstet Gynecol 1985;66(6):816–20.
7. TeamSTEPPS National implementation [cited 2011 December 30]. Available at: http://teamstepps.ahrq.gov/. Accessed December 30, 2011.
8. Lindegren ML, Byers RH Jr, Thomas P, et al. Trends in perinatal transmission of HIV/AIDS in the United States. JAMA 1999;282(6):531–8.
9. Maryland AAD. [cited 2010 December 1]. Available at: www.dhmh.state.md.us/AIDS. Accessed December 1, 2010.
10. Mighty H, Kriebs J. Legal issues in obstetrics and gynecology. In: Reese EA, Barbieri RL, editors. Obstetrics and gynecology: the essentials of clinical care. Stuttgart (Germany): Thieme; 2010. p. 527–32.

11. Iqbal SN, Kriebs J, Harman C, et al. Predictors of fetal growth in maternal HIV disease. Am J Perinatol 2010;27(7):517–23.
12. Iqbal S, Kriebs J, Harman C, et al. Protease inhibitor therapy and fetal growth potential in HIV-positive women. Am J Perinatol 2008;25(6):335–9.
13. Miller J, Dangel A, Fahey J, et al. Feasibility of continuous glucose monitoring in labor. Am J Obstet Gynecol 2009;201(Suppl 6):S108.
14. Kasdaglis T, Kriebs J, Harman C, et al. Pregnancy in perinatally infected HIV patients: are outcomes any different? Am J Obstet Gynecol 2008;199:SA6 S147.
15. Iqbal S, Harman C, Alger L, et al. Predictors of fetal growth restriction (FGR) in maternal HIV disease. Am J Obstet Gynecol 2007;197(6 Suppl 1). S94.
16. Baschat A, Butkowski R, Kush M, et al. Fetal growth potential in HIV-positive patients. Am J Obstet Gynecol 2003;189(6 Suppl 1):S217.
17. Fahey JO, Mighty HE. Shoulder dystocia: using simulation to train providers and teams. J Perinat Neonatal Nurs 2008;22(2):114–22.
18. Dyachenko A, Ciampi A, Fahey J, et al. Prediction of risk for shoulder dystocia with neonatal injury. Am J Obstet Gynecol 2006;195:1544–9.
19. Mighty HE, Fahey J. Obesity and pregnancy complications. Curr Diab Rep 2007; 7:289–94.
20. Mighty HE, Fahey JO. Clinical ethics in obstetrics and gynecology. In: Reece AE, Barbieri RL, editors. Obstetrics and gynecology: the essential of clinical care. New York: Thieme; 2010. p. 517–26.

# Working Toward a Common Goal

## A Collaborative Obstetrics and Gynecology Practice

Nicole Marshall, CNM, NP, MS, Sarah Egan, CNM, MS*, Christina Flores, MD, Abbe Kirsch, CNM, MS, Ruth Mankoff, CNM, MS, Melissa Resnick, CNM, MS

**KEYWORDS**

• Obstetrics • Gynecology • Collaboration • Health care reform

**KEY POINTS**

- Bronx-Lebanon Hospital Center's Obstetrics and Gynecology Department can be used as a model for delivery of routine and specialty women's health care.
- Collaborative practice among physicians and midwives allows patients to benefit from the strengths of both disciplines.
- In conjunction with physician colleagues, midwifery is an ideal cost-effective option for expanding safe obstetric and gynecologic care to high-risk women.

## INTRODUCTION

Using a collaborative model of care between obstetrics/gynecology attending physicians, midwives, physician assistants, and residents has encouraged the providers of the Bronx-Lebanon Hospital Center (BLHC) to approach patient care with a common goal always in mind: to provide high-quality, specialized patient care to an underserved community. This article describes the evolution of this model and its current approach to collaboration in serving this community.

BLHC is the largest voluntary, not-for-profit health care system serving South and Central Bronx, New York, a densely populated urban area. The immediate surrounding neighborhood is predominantly low-income ($16,496 median per capita) and comprises minorities (62% Hispanic; 35% African/African American) numbering more than 762,600 people.[1] This area has the highest rates of poverty, imprisonment, and lack of education in New York City and has been designated as a Health Professional Shortage/Medically Underserved Area by the US Department of Health and Human Services.[2]

Bronx County has a disproportionately high rate of many leading health indicators. For instance, compared with the rest of the country, the rate of low-birth-weight babies (<2500 g) is nearly 25% higher, adolescent pregnancies (ages 15–17 years)

Department of OB/GYN, Bronx-Lebanon Hospital Center, 1650 Grand Concourse, Bronx, NY 10457, USA
* Corresponding author.
*E-mail address:* sarahegancnm@gmail.com

Obstet Gynecol Clin N Am 39 (2012) 373–382
http://dx.doi.org/10.1016/j.ogc.2012.05.006
obgyn.theclinics.com

are almost double, diabetes in adults is higher by approximately 30%, and new human immunodeficiency virus (HIV) diagnoses (per 100,000) are triple.[3,4] Many patients are new immigrants from the Caribbean, Latin America, West Africa, and the Indian subcontinent. More than half do not speak English at home,[1] relying on their family, friends, or community services to help them negotiate life in this country.

For many women in this immigrant population, pregnancy or childbirth is the first point of contact with the United States health care system. On any given day, providers can be found speaking English, Spanish, French, or Arabic. Translator phones allow communication in many other languages, such as Twi, Bengali, Soninke, and Bambara.

The BLHC Obstetrics and Gynecology Department comprises 20 attending physicians, 17 residents, 17 midwives, and 3 physician assistants. The midwifery department, consisting of certified nurse midwives as well as certified midwives, has more than doubled in size during the past decade. Together, 70,000 outpatient visits are conducted annually. Each year, an average of 9000 patients are triaged on the labor floor and approximately 3,000 births are attended. Dedication, partnership, and excellent teamwork are the backbone of the department. Without these key elements, such high-quality medical care could not be offered to this large number of women.

## OUR HISTORY

A new chairman was appointed to the Department of Obstetrics and Gynecology at BLHC in 1998. Having worked with midwives during his residency and as a junior attending physician, he saw an opportunity to foster the growth of a midwifery service. His commitment to action helped to counter initial resistance to the presence of midwives by educating staff about the scope and principles of midwifery practice and how these both overlapped with and differed from the traditional medical model.

Midwifery in New York State is defined as, “the management of normal pregnancies, childbirth and postpartum care, as well as primary preventive reproductive health care of essentially healthy women, and shall include newborn evaluation, resuscitation and referral for infants.”[5] Licensed midwives in New York have full prescriptive authority, including Drug Enforcement Administration numbers and the ability to practice independently.[5]

The original service began with 3 midwives working in the clinic and on the labor and delivery unit. In the ambulatory setting, independent midwifery care was quickly accepted. The Director of Midwives was also appointed Director of the Women’s Health Center (the main hospital outpatient clinic) where she worked closely with the Obstetrics/Gynecology Department Chairman to ensure the practice compliance required by the Joint Commission, Medicaid/Medicare, and various managed care organizations. As the clinic responsibilities increased, an obstetrician/gynecologist physician was appointed Codirector, working in collaboration with the Midwifery Director. In time, the midwifery presence has increased and now has 17 midwives, with practice experience ranging from recent graduates to those with more than 30 years of experience. As the service grew, their roles have become more varied, both in the inpatient and outpatient settings.

## OUTPATIENT SERVICES

The Women’s Health Center offers both routine obstetric and gynecologic care and access to specialists, including maternal-fetal medicine, urologic gynecology, colposcopy, gynecologic oncology, reproductive endocrinology, termination of pregnancy, and adolescent services with group prenatal care. This extensive network of services in 1 physical location is convenient for patients, and also allows ease of consultation and collaboration among the provider network. It reduces duplication of services, resulting in more cost-effective care. The Comprehensive Care Center, which follows patients with HIV/acquired immune deficiency syndrome (AIDS), is the only obstetric or gynecologic service not provided at this location.

New patients scheduled for routine care at BLHC are randomly given an appointment with the next available provider, either a physician or a midwife. To ensure continuity of care, patients are encouraged to see the same provider throughout their pregnancy. However, a midwifery patient is sometimes transferred to physician care because of the high-risk nature of her pregnancy or health condition. At times, a patient changes providers based on language or cultural needs.

As independent clinicians, the midwives at BLHC provide the full scope women's health care, including birth attendance and outpatient reproductive care, with a physician always available for consultation. In our large multispecialty collaborative model, midwives have the unique opportunity to expand their scope of practice and obtain skills beyond that of their core competencies, and patients have the opportunity to continue to receive midwifery care even in specialty clinics, such as in high-risk pregnancy, abortion, colposcopy, and infectious disease.

## FAMILY PLANNING/TERMINATION OF PREGNANCY CLINIC

In 2008, Bronx County had the highest abortion ratio (number of induced abortions per 1000 live births) in New York State (903.8).[6] To meet this need, BLHC offers termination of pregnancy in accordance with New York State law, up to the legal limit of 23 6/7 weeks' gestation. Patients are referred from clinics and private offices from New York City, neighboring states, and occasionally from countries with more restrictive abortion laws. A midwife performs a complete history, physical examination, and ultrasound, and prepares the patient for the procedure, including inserting cervical dilators and prescribing cervical ripening agents. Counseling services are paramount, because indications for late termination of pregnancy often include fetal anomalies, maternal comorbidities, and significant social stressors. The procedure is performed by a physician, but the midwife and physician work closely together in the patient's care. Their collaboration is crucial, particularly in late gestations. Our patients often have significant obstetric and/or medical histories, including multiple prior cesareans, placental abnormalities, morbid obesity, poorly controlled hypertension, or diabetes. The midwife and physician recently jointly developed a protocol for immediate intrauterine device placement after termination. All providers extensively counsel patients regarding contraceptive options. This teamwork allows the women of the Bronx to benefit from a broad array of family planning options, potentially resulting in a decrease in the need for elective abortion services.

## CENTER FOR COMPREHENSIVE CARE (HIV SERVICES)

In 2008, there were 9134 women living with HIV/AIDS in the Bronx; more than 96% are women of color.[7] Citywide, the highest proportion of new female HIV diagnoses is in the Bronx, with heterosexual intercourse as the predominant risk factor.[8] Since the onset of the epidemic in New York City, BLHC has been a leader in providing care and services to HIV-infected individuals and their families. The BLHC Department of Obstetrics and Gynecology has successfully developed and implemented numerous programs targeting HIV-positive and high-risk women and men, including: Prevention Services for Women (PSW), Prevention and Related Services for Women (PRSW),

Family-Centered Health Care Services (FCC) since 2003, and Community Action for Prenatal Care Initiative (Bronx CAPC), a coalition of 34 agencies.

All women entering prenatal care at our hospital are tested for HIV, in accordance with New York State law. Any woman identified as HIV-positive is counseled by a trained HIV counselor, escorted to the Comprehensive Care Center, and introduced immediately to the midwife (Director of Women's HIV Services) and/or the maternal-fetal medicine physician (Codirector). The patient's prenatal care begins on the same day. Both the midwife and physician are HIV specialists, as designated by the New York State AIDS Institute. These providers maintain their HIV specialist designation by completing HIV-related continuing education on an ongoing basis. Antiretroviral therapy during pregnancy is comanaged by the midwife, physician, and each patient's primary HIV provider. Women with additional comorbidities or complicated obstetric histories are managed solely by the perinatologist. Routine gynecologic care, including preconception counseling for infected women and their partners, contraception, STD screening, and colposcopy, are also provided on-site by the midwife. The physician does not provide inpatient care, making the midwife the main point of contact for the continuity of care for HIV-infected women during any obstetric admission.

Multidisciplinary case conferences attended by the medical and case management teams, as well as by Bronx CAPC, are held at least twice monthly. Pregnant and newborn clients are discussed at each meeting, as are families in crisis. Every family is discussed at least once every 180 days. The case management team maintains lists of internal and community resources that provide supportive and risk-reduction services. This branch of the Department of Obstetrics and Gynecology is the lead agency for Bronx CAPC, which uses outreach workers specially trained to engage the most difficult-to-reach women, including women recently discharged from the New York City Department of Corrections. This family-centered model ensures the collaboration of all members of the health care team.

## HIGH-RISK PREGNANCY CLINIC

The high-risk obstetrics clinic is staffed by a perinatologist, an attending physician, 2 midwives, a physician assistant, and 2 to 3 obstetric residents. Each patient is cared for by the resident, midwife, or physician assistant, and then the case is reviewed with the perinatologist or attending physician before the patient's discharge from the clinic. The multiple providers in this model provide a variety of benefits to the patients, the individual providers, and our department as a whole.

Patients can request a specific provider, based on a prior relationship, language, or other cultural need, and often they seek out a midwife or physician assistant who is present at every clinic session. Residents rotate through the clinic, and thus are not able to provide true continuity of care in the clinic for the duration of the pregnancy; however, patients sometimes try to see the same 2 or 3 residents during their pregnancy. This model enables the provider to continue with the plan of care rather than having to start again with a complex history at each visit, and each chart is reviewed by 1 of the same 3 attending physicians at every clinic session. High-risk pregnancies also offer a unique opportunity for clinicians to provide education and empower women to better care for themselves and their families, especially when social or psychiatric issues are present. The collaboration among the providers results in maximizing both the medical and psychosocial care of our most complicated patients.

For the providers, involvement in the high-risk clinic with close collaboration with maternal-fetal medicine means gaining the knowledge and experience to manage a multitude of complications. The relationships between the midwives and physicians are built on mutual respect, with the common goal of trying to provide the best care for the patient. This policy carries over into inpatient care, where midwives comanage more complicated patients instead of referring them solely for physician management. The residents benefit by gaining confidence in counseling and caring for the profound psychosocial needs of these patients, rather than concentrating exclusively on their medical care.

Our department as a whole has benefitted from the close working relationships among the midwives serving on the high-risk team, physician assistants, residents, and the attending physicians. Mutual respect results in greater professionalism, trust, and collegiality.

## ADOLESCENT SERVICES

The Women's Health Center offers specialized services to women up to 21 years of age, focusing intensively on education and counseling. For a period of 1 year beginning in 2008, the department participated in Integrating Prenatal Care to Reduce HIV/STDs Among Teens: A Translational Study, sponsored by Yale University, Clinical Directors Network and the Centering Healthcare Institute. This study was funded by the National Institute of Health.[9] As 1 of 14 sites in New York City, the Centering Pregnancy model of group prenatal care was launched in the Women's Health Center.[10] The group model of care continues, currently allowing adolescent patients to choose between group or individualized care in the teen clinic. Centering Pregnancy groups are facilitated by midwives alongside a social worker or registered nurse. The specialty clinic offers individualized care to young women age 12 to 21 years, and is staffed by 3 midwives. Resident physicians, both obstetric and pediatric, also work at this clinic during their elective rotation.

## COMMUNITY HEALTH CENTERS

BLHC has 5 satellite clinics that provide obstetric and gynecologic services. One is staffed exclusively by attending physicians, whereas the others are solely staffed by midwives. Physician consultation is always available, and patients can be referred to the Women's Health Center as needed, where additional specialty services are offered.

## INPATIENT: CHANGES OVER TIME

In contrast with the relative ease of the integration of midwives in the outpatient setting, changes in the labor and delivery came more slowly. Twelve years ago, all births, regardless of level of acuity, were generally treated with the same high level of intervention. Women were prohibited from ambulating in labor and rushed to the delivery room just before crowning; the entire labor floor had the feeling of an intensive care unit. Obstetricians by training and habit were inclined to intervene more often than the midwives, who were attempting to follow the midwifery protocol for the management of normal labor.

Reconstruction of the labor floor was the perfect opportunity for change: bath tubs or showers were installed in all labor-delivery-recovery rooms (LDRs), and ambulation, intermittent fetal heart rate monitoring, and hydrotherapy for labor and birth became accepted and encouraged. The renovated unit has a 4-bed triage area, 7 LDRs, 2 operating rooms, and a 4-bed recovery room.

Labor and delivery is now staffed by 4 residents, 1 midwife, and 1 attending physician. In 2009, there were 2708 births; the cesarean rate was 34.5%, and the rate of successful vaginal birth after cesarean (VBAC) was 53%. Midwives attended 18%

of all vaginal births. Hydrotherapy and/or water birth is available for appropriate candidates.

Most patients who present to triage are from the BLHC network. About 20% of women come from other hospitals or have not had any prenatal care. BLHC is also a transfer hospital for a local freestanding birthing center.

During their pregnancies, women who received prenatal care with the BLHC midwives are designated prenatally as midwife patients with a sticker on their so-called Pregnancy Passport (a card containing obstetric information). These women are ideally evaluated in triage, and, if admitted, managed and delivered by a midwife. The attending physician is updated about the progress of all patients and is immediately available for consultation or for situations that require instrumental or cesarean delivery. Low-risk women who develop complications during labor are comanaged by the physician and midwife. Women who were high risk in their pregnancy but at the time of delivery are low risk, such as women with a history of preterm delivery currently laboring with a full-term pregnancy, may be managed by a midwife. In cases that are less clearly defined, the decision is made on a case-by-case basis, according to the comfort levels and degrees of experience among the on-call team.

In addition to triage and labor management duties, all residents and midwives precept medical students, family practice, and emergency room residents during their obstetric rotation, and midwifery students. The antepartum service is covered by a monthly rotating attending physician, the obstetric team of residents for that quarter, and a physician assistant. The midwives conduct social rounds of their own patients. Midwives are responsible for the postpartum care and discharge of the women delivered by the midwives. This responsibility includes those low-risk patients from other hospitals who were assigned for midwifery management on presentation to labor and delivery. The residents conduct rounds of the women delivered by physicians, as well as the postoperative patients. Often the midwife provides breastfeeding assistance regardless of mode of delivery. Follow-up after discharge is usually with the provider who saw the patient prenatally, allowing for continuity of care.

All pregnant patients at BLHC are made aware of the Pregnancy Hotline, a 24-hour number available for any questions or concerns. The hotline connects the patient to the labor floor, where residents or midwives answer the call.

## INTERDISCIPLINARY EDUCATION

Interdisciplinary education is an important facet of collaborative practice. All members of the department attend weekly grand rounds. At these meetings, a specific topic is presented, cases are reviewed, and ways to improve practice outcomes are analyzed. Multidisciplinary lecturers at these educational rounds include physicians, nurses, midwives, and other professionals.

Beginning in 2007, the department invested a significant amount of time and revenue into Team Performance Plus, a risk-reduction program. This model was developed in partnership with, and taught by, award-winning trainers from Beth Israel Deaconess Medical Center in Boston (MA), as an interdisciplinary training program for obstetric units, applying concepts of crew resource management used by commercial and military flight teams.[11] The goal is to reduce morbidity and mortality caused by preventable medical errors or poor communication. Our approach involves creating an interdisciplinary core team, contingency team, and coordinating team for every shift. Any member of the unit can call for a team meeting to address concerns, gather patient information, or create a management plan. Removing the hierarchical structure from labor and delivery empowers all staff members to address concerns that could potentially benefit patient safety. Yearly refresher courses are required of all staff, and all new staff members are trained in the program as part of the orientation process.

In addition to team training, all providers have completed a mandated Fetal Heart Rate Monitoring Interpretation and Intrapartum Management course, cosponsored by FOJP Service Corporation, Risk Management Advisors, and Mount Sinai School of Medicine. This course ensures that all midwives, nurses, and physicians on labor and delivery are using the same standardized terminology, increasing the ease of communication and management decisions among all clinical staff. As with team training, biannual refresher courses are mandated, and ongoing courses are available for new staff.

Continuing education is mandatory for reappointment to the medical staff of BLHC. Often physicians and midwives attend the same conferences, facilitating the exchange of ideas. Other interdisciplinary educational opportunities in our department include emergency drills such as best management of shoulder dystocia, eclampsia, and maternal hemorrhage.

BLHC is a clinical site for obstetric and gynecologic clerkships for several medical schools. Midwives present the basics of normal labor and birth as the students' first exposure to obstetrics. The midwives and physicians share responsibility for the students, both in the clinic and on the labor floor. These students are offered a unique opportunity to be part of a true interdisciplinary team, and leave our site with a greater appreciation for the positive impact collaborative practice can have on patient care.

BLHC is a National Health Service Corps (NHSC) site. This federal program offers student loan repayment in reciprocation for their primary care service for the underserved. Both midwives and obstetrician/gynecologists attending physicians are eligible to receive this grant. Recipients are encouraged to attend lectures and conferences that address the specific issues related to working with an underserved population. Through the NHSC program, BLHC is able to attract motivated, passionate clinicians who are committed to best practices in obstetric and gynecologic care.

## FUTURE ENDEAVORS

As a department, we hope to safely decrease our cesarean section rate and increase our rate of successful VBACs, in alignment with the goals of Healthy People 2020.[12] Increasing the midwifery presence on labor and delivery, as well as continuing midwifery involvement in medical student and resident education, will result in a greater appreciation of physiologic labor and birth, potentially decreasing early labor admissions and thus decreasing surgical intervention for failure to progress.

The whirlpool tubs available on our labor and delivery unit are unique among the hospitals in New York City. The only providers with any experience caring for women using hydrotherapy in labor are currently the midwives, and, although the tubs are featured prominently in the marketing for the obstetric services at BLHC, if a midwife is not available on the labor floor or if the unit is busy, hydrotherapy is not an option. Further education is needed for our resident and nursing staff on intermittent fetal heart rate auscultation and how to safely care for women who choose to use tubs during labor and birth.

Midwives in many other hospitals are included as part of the surgical team on labor and delivery as a first assistant on cesarean sections. At BLHC, there is a potential to increase the involvement of the midwives as surgical assistants, and this will be explored in the future.

The collaborative practice in our termination of pregnancy clinic has been increasing in the last few years. Although residents are beginning to rotate through this specialty and receive training from the midwife in preprocedure preparation, future practice changes could add the provision of medical abortion services by the midwives.

The adolescent services at BLHC are well used by the community. Involving resident and attending physicians in formal training in Centering Pregnancy group prenatal care would increase their participation. All women who are expecting their first baby could benefit from group prenatal care, with a strong focus on education and self-empowerment.

The HIV services for women are a highly regarded component of the department. In the near future, rapid testing will be available for all patients, providing same-day counseling and results. In addition, a walk-in referral clinic is being planned for the partners of all women who are diagnosed with a sexually transmitted infection, allowing diagnosis and treatment in a timely fashion.

## COLLABORATION: A PHYSICIAN'S PERSPECTIVE

My initial exposure to midwives began when I accepted my first job at BLHC after residency training. I trained at a community hospital in Long Island (NY), where my only comanaged patient experience was with physicians of other disciplines. After learning of the large midwifery service, but before starting work at BLHC, I found it difficult to visualize this collaborative model; however, I value interdisciplinary care, so I was excited to see how this practice design would operate.

Many of the midwives at BLHC have numerous years of experience. I found that reassuring as a new attending in a new environment. I quickly became comfortable with the midwives both professionally and personally. It became evident that their genuine compassion was not just for their patients but also for their coworkers and ancillary staff. I found it easy to develop trust, which is key for successful patient care. I soon realized that the midwives' philosophy aligned with my own: the patient is priority number 1. The more I work with the midwives, the more confidence I gain in their management decisions.

The midwives and physicians at BLHC are true interdisciplinary partners. We work side by side in the clinic setting and in tandem on the labor floor. There is always 1 midwife assigned to labor and delivery, giving them the opportunity to continue the care with the obstetric patients they follow in the clinic. They triage patients, manage them in labor, and ultimately deliver their own patients. Continuity of care is encouraged at BLHC, and, through this model, we have seen a positive difference in patient satisfaction. Midwives and physicians, through frequent communication, ensure that all providers involved in a patient's care are kept abreast, which is important for many reasons; for example, a midwife's patient may need a cesarean section, and the physician performing the surgery is aware and involved in the case from the beginning.

Also, case presentations and discussions with another provider are helpful in that they create a natural system of checks and balances. Because patient safety is a priority at BLHC, this interdisciplinary system adds to a comprehensive care model and ultimately reduces medical errors, leading to better outcomes.

I continue to have positive experiences with the midwives both in the outpatient setting and on the labor floor. One event in particular inspired me to be one of the authors of this article. At BLHC, hydrotherapy is offered for labor and birth. Many of the physicians were not trained in water births; thus, we rely on the midwives in these situations to facilitate the patient's plan for birth. I was fortunate to be on call one night with a midwife when a patient in labor arrived and requested to have a tub birth. I was happy to collaborate with the midwife to successfully accommodate the patient's wishes. The midwife followed the patient through a normal labor progression. At the time of delivery, the patient had her support people around her, the midwife was compassionately supporting her with every push, and this culminated in one of the most graceful, serene, controlled deliveries I have ever seen. Once the baby was delivered, the midwife placed the baby on the patient's breast immediately. It was the most amazing experience that the patient, the patient's family, and I had ever witnessed. It made me appreciate even more the different skills the midwives bring to this interdisciplinary practice.

The midwives and physicians collaborate not only in practice but also in education. This collaboration is especially apparent with our 17 residents. That July, when I started as an intern in my residency program, I remember feeling grateful that anyone would help me figure out what I needed to do and how to do it. It was an anxious time for me. At BLHC, when the new interns start on labor and delivery, the midwives teach them in multiple ways: everything from sonograms to cervical examinations. They also teach them how to evaluate patients who come through triage.

The medical students who rotate with us are able to see different management styles and get a lot of hands-on experience with the midwives. In my experience, most of the midwives at BLHC are interested in teaching, creating a work environment in which residents and students can express their concerns and ask questions without anxiety or stress. The role the midwives play in education is as important as that of the attending physicians. This interdisciplinary paradigm enhances the educational setting at our hospital, increasing both patient safety and provider satisfaction.

There are many misconceptions about supposed management conflicts and power struggles in obstetric care. I have never experienced these issues with the group practice of physicians and midwives at BLHC. When patient care and education are the top priorities in a community hospital similar to ours, the work atmosphere can be harmonious as the staff strive toward a common goal.

## SUMMARY

The South Bronx has a treasure in the Obstetrics and Gynecology Department at BLHC. The combination of the knowledge, expertise, passion, and energy of its providers offers a superior experience for patients and their families. We plan to continue to grow our practice, increasing the opportunities to build relationships among all of our clinicians. The respect and collaborative spirit among our team is one that other hospitals would benefit from emulating, and one that will continue to result in compassionate, sensitive care for the women of the Bronx.

## REFERENCES


1. US Census, 2005–2007 American Community Survey 3-Year Estimates.
2. Women's HIV Collaborative of New York. Women Living with HIV and AIDS in NYC: a mapping project and literature review, 2008.
3. New York State indicators for tracking public health priority areas. Available at: http://www.health.state.ny.us/prevention/prevention_agenda/indicators/county/bronx.htm. Accessed January 9, 2011.
4. The World Health Organization Department of Making Pregnancy Safer. Available at: http://www.who.int/making_pregnancy_safer/documents/who_frh_msm_9624/en. Accessed January 10, 2011.
5. NYS Office of Professions. Available at: http://www.op.nysed.gov/prof/midwife. Accessed January 5, 2011.

6. NYS Office of Health Vital Statistics. Available at: http://www.health.state.ny.us/nysdoh/vital/_statistics/2008/table22.htm. Accessed January 20, 2011.
7. NYC DOHMH-HIV Epidemiology and Field Services Program, 2008 Surveillance Tables.
8. NYC DOHMH-HIV Epidemiology and Field Services Program, HIV/AIDS among females 2008, slides.
9. National Institute of Health. Available at: http://clinicaltrials.gov/ct2/show/NCT00628771. Accessed January 8, 2011.
10. Rising SS, Kennedy HP, Klima C. Redesigning prenatal care through Centering-Pregnancy. J Midwifery Womens Health 2004;49(5):398–404.
11. Mann S, Marcus R, Sachs B. Lessons from the cockpit: how team training can reduce errors on L&D. Contemp Ob Gyn 2006.
12. Healthy People 2020. Available at: http://www.healthypeople.gov/hp2020. Accessed January 10, 2011.

# Collaborative Maternity Care

## Three Decades of Success at Dartmouth-Hitchcock Medical Center

Miriam N. Cordell, MS, CNM[a], Tina C. Foster, MD, MPH, MS[b], Emily R. Baker, MD[c], Barbara Fildes, MS, CNM[d,*]

**KEYWORDS**

- Collaborative practice • Maternity • Women's health
- Dartmouth-Hitchcock Medical Center

**KEY POINT**

- Successful collaborative practice is an evolving process linked to mission, vision, and goals in providing care.

## INTRODUCTION

The word colLABORative indicates that hard work is involved (and perhaps that those who care for women around the time of birth are especially suited for such practice). However, more than just persistence and effort is required. Courage is essential, as exemplified by the efforts of the bold early adopters at Dartmouth-Hitchcock Medical Center (DHMC), who responded to the community's needs by offering a new type of care that was woman centered. Underlying that hard work and willingness to take risks are deeper values that cannot simply be encompassed under the heading of a practice model. Shared aims, trust, and respect are the underpinnings of success at Dartmouth, and, we suspect, elsewhere. Without these, we could not achieve genuine

All work was performed at Dartmouth-Hitchcock Medical Center.
The authors have no disclosures of financial support.
[a] Division of Nurse-Midwives and Practitioners, Department of Obstetrics and Gynecology, Dartmouth-Hitchcock Medical Center, Dartmouth Medical School, One Medical Center Drive, Lebanon, NH 03756, USA; [b] Division of General Obstetrics and Gynecology, Dartmouth-Hitchcock Medical Center, Dartmouth Medical School, One Medical Center Drive, Lebanon, NH 03756, USA; [c] Division of Maternal-Fetal Medicine, Department of Obstetrics and Gynecology, Dartmouth-Hitchcock Medical Center, Dartmouth Medical School, One Medical Center Drive, Lebanon, NH 03756, USA; [d] Regional Obstetrics Improvement, New England Alliance for Health at Dartmouth-Hitchcock Medical Center, Dartmouth Medical School, One Medical Center Drive, Lebanon, NH 03756, USA
* Corresponding author.
*E-mail address:* barbara.fildes@hitchcock.org

Obstet Gynecol Clin N Am 39 (2012) 383–398
http://dx.doi.org/10.1016/j.ogc.2012.05.007 **obgyn.theclinics.com**
0889-8545/12/$ – see front matter 

collaboration, nor could we benefit from the endless opportunities to learn from each other. Ongoing inquiry and dialogue among collaborators is crucial, as is ongoing engagement with the ultimate beneficiaries (and judges) of our care: the women in our care. This article describes the development of our collaborative practice, as well as the questions we have confronted (and continue to confront). It shares some of the joy that our providers, learners, and patients have experienced during the last 3 decades.

### *Background for Initiation of Collaborative Practice*

Collaborative practice at DHMC began with a desire on the part of women in the community to modify the care they were receiving. This desire occurred at a time when an all-male group of obstetrician-gynecologists (OB/GYNs), looking at changes taking place nationally and listening to women locally, sought to recruit more female colleagues to the department. These physicians broke new ground in the 1970s when they prepared 2 nurses to become OB/GYN nurse practitioners, a new role with little regulation or oversight of education. This experiment proved successful in the outpatient practice and laid the groundwork for the future collaborative practice with nurse-midwives. In the early 1980s, a survey was sent to women who had received maternity care at DHMC asking what they would like to see changed. Responses were consistent: women wanted more female providers; continuity of care as they moved through pregnancy, birth, and parenting; and more time with providers. George Little, MD (Doctor of Medicine), a neonatologist, and Jack Dodds, MD, an OB/GYN, saw nurse-midwifery as a potential solution.

After reading about nurse-midwifery and taking field trips to explore practices, these department leaders recruited Charlotte Houde-Quimby, a certified nurse-midwife (CNM), from a private practice in New Haven, Connecticut, as the first Director of the Nurse-Midwifery Service. The decision was made to hire 3 additional CNMs who were exceptional clinicians and possessed master's degrees, which was not the standard at the time. In doing so, the department was able to negotiate faculty appointments for these first 4 nurse-midwives at Dartmouth Medical School, thereby providing another solid piece in the foundation of the collaborative practice. By 1983, the public embraced the newly formed Nurse-Midwifery Service and women were traveling long distances to receive their care at Dartmouth-Hitchcock.

## CHALLENGES AND SOLUTIONS: FIRST DECADE 1983 TO 1993

Physicians and CNMs have practiced collaboratively at DHMC for nearly 30 years. Each decade brought challenges and opportunities that changed their practice. Their ability to respond to dynamic clinical, economic, and legal conditions while maintaining focus on the women they serve has maintained and grown the collaborative practice.

Collaborative practice is not likely to be sustainable in settings in which it is continually challenged or overtly opposed by nurses and physicians. Before CNMs came to Dartmouth-Hitchcock, the inpatient registered nurses (RNs) worked with a small group of obstetricians on a busy unit without obstetrics residents. They feared the loss of their identity and diminishing roles for them once the CNMs arrived. In response, the CNMs spent time with the nurses to learn about how they worked and to discern how the unit operated, well in advance of admitting their first patients in 1983. Because the CNMs had been labor and delivery nurses, they understood and addressed the fears expressed by the nursing staff. Grand Rounds was used as a forum to present a collaborative model of MD-CNM-RN partnership. Working side by side, day by day proved to be the most effective means of showing that MDs, CNMs, and RNs are all essential and valued members of the team.

The generalist OB/GYNs had worked with nurse practitioners in the outpatient setting for many years and expressed few worries. One senior physician informed his patients that he needed to have major surgery and that the CNMs would be taking care of them during his medical leave. This arrangement afforded the CNMs the opportunity to conduct a substantial number of births shortly after their arrival. Another physician, considered to be an exceptional clinician, had done his residency at Yale and contacted physician colleagues there to discuss their work with the new CNM Director. Receiving reassurance, he asked to observe her conduct some births. After doing so, he publicly supported the collaborative practice and served as teacher and mentor for CNMs in the coming decades. The Clerkship Director invited the CNMs into medical education from the earliest days and valued their creative teaching strategies. The maternal-fetal medicine (MFM) physicians worked to keep women with the Nurse-Midwifery Service whenever possible and modeled comanagement of pregnancy complications. The Department Chair was available for brainstorming as soon as a problem arose.

There was initial resistance from anesthesia personnel to responding when called by the CNMs, and this was resolved in a leadership meeting. When ultrasound and laboratory requests signed by CNMs were refused, the CNMs sent several women to an outside facility that willingly provided these services. The CNMs then presented this to radiology and laboratory leadership and the matter was resolved. A local childbirth educator became a credible advocate for the new model of care with local families. CNMs presented their model to local community groups. The CNMs acknowledged that the strong foundation for collaborative practice at DHMC was constructed by MDs who saw change coming, listened to women, and put something different in place than what they had been offering. The CNMs showed endurance, resourcefulness, and clinical acumen and skill as they provided uninterrupted coverage for their caseload, every day and every night. Uninterrupted coverage became a hallmark of this practice. With grace, the CNMs challenged clinical practices that were common in the 1980s and showed safe alternatives to traditional obstetric procedures such as episiotomy. Their presence changed practice and culture.

As the 1990s approached, the practice was acclaimed in the community and served families from all walks of life, including nurses, physicians, and others who had, years before, challenged the move away from the traditional model of care. A decision was made to relocate the CNMs to a new community health center 1.6 km from the medical center. The goal was to provide an office environment outside the busy medical center that was better suited to healthy, young families, and to practice in proximity with physicians in the Department of Community and Family Medicine, many of whom did not wish to provide obstetric and gynecologic care. As the first decade of collaborative practice drew to a close, the experiment of moving the CNMs away from their home department was in full swing; a new reimbursement concept, managed care, was spotted on the horizon; competition from community hospitals was increasing; and the trusted CNM and MD leaders who founded the practice were moving on to the next stage of their careers.

## CHALLENGES AND SOLUTIONS: SECOND DECADE 1993 TO 2003

The second decade was one of growth by design, punctuated by frequent and disparate changes in the practice environment, few of which could have been anticipated. By the end of the decade, the Division of Midwives and OB/GYN nurse practitioners in the newly organized Department of Obstetrics and Gynecology was larger than the entire department had been when the CNMs and MDs began their collaborative practice. A new CNM Director was in place; a lengthy search for Department Chair had been accomplished; a full complement of subspecialist physicians had been recruited; an application for a new OB/GYN residency was approved by the Residency Review Committee (RRC); the Clinical Information System, a precursor of electronic medical records (EMRs), was becoming the norm; advanced practice registered nurse (APRN) roles were created to support the subspecialists; an Administrative Director and Practice Manager were embedded in the department; routine coding and billing seemed to have evolved into a foreign language; and the gender mix of the department was altered as young, female physicians joined the ranks. Organizational leadership became focused on productivity, profitability, and compliance.

Attention was focused on a new academic discipline established by local colleagues to explore clinical practice, health policy, and health care delivery systems. That group moved to the forefront of the national health care debate a decade later as The Dartmouth Institute for Health Policy and Clinical Practice, now recognized as a leading contributor to the discussion about how best to deliver care in the United States. The CNMs and MDs began to understand that this new science in outcomes would forever change how their care would be evaluated.

During this time, the CNMs feared loss of identity and diminishing roles. They stayed focused clinically, leading the way in the 1990s for improvements in care related to postpartum length of stay, postpartum depression, cervical ripening, hydrotherapy, menopause, and vaginal birth after cesarean (VBAC). Along with anesthesia colleagues, they framed the epidural debate in a way that unified the CNMs, RNs, and MDs, regardless of personal beliefs, and helped them guide the women in their care. They expanded their commitment to rural women by assuming primary responsibility for 4 distant sites where they conducted clinics and coordinated care at the medical center. The CNMs and MDs together advocated for dental services and mental health care for pregnant women who were uninsured or covered by Medicaid. CNMs became a mainstay in the care for a growing number of victims of sexual and domestic violence. Balancing this with other clinical demands became overwhelming and the CNMs advocated for establishment of a Sexual Assault Nurse Examiner (SANE) program and served as initial trainers.

CNMs continued to attend approximately half the low-risk births at the medical center, which represented about one-third of the total obstetric volume; taught pelvic examination skills with second-year medical students; participated in didactic and clinical teaching with third-year medical students; and educated student nurse-midwives from a variety of universities.

Having the CNMs share office space and support staff with Family Practice but remain financially and clinically accountable to OB/GYN was increasingly confusing for the community and burdensome for the staff. A decision was made to gradually phase the CNMs back into the Department of Obstetrics/Gynecology and dedicated secretarial, nursing, and phone triage support was put in place. To improve access for pregnant women, the CNMs gently transitioned women to gynecology care with MD or APRN colleagues, modified schedule templates, conducted a year-long group prenatal care pilot project based on new work called CenteringPregnancy, and reentered the world of childbirth education. The renewed CNM focus on the care of pregnant women had positive consequences as the next round of changes occurred.

With the establishment of the Division of Maternal-Fetal Medicine and the arrival of the first class of residents, there needed to be a reevaluation of how CNMs would fit into the emerging model. The CNM and MD leaders adopted fresh thinking and made decisions about the collaborative practice after collecting data from the American College of Nurse-Midwives (ACNM), the Midwifery Business Institute, the American College of Obstetricians and Gynecologists (ACOG), other academic practices, and the growing number of MD/APRN practices within DHMC.

The Nurse-Midwifery Service remained intact and continued to provide uninterrupted care for a discrete caseload of women, as a component of the new Division of Midwives and Nurse Practitioners. All consultation, comanagement, and referral would take place with MFM MDs and a weekly consult meeting included all CNMs, a nurse, and an appointment secretary. This system reduced variation in clinical practice and offered women improved continuity of care at a time when the obstetric caseload was becoming more complex. This steady MFM/CNM partnership helped women feel safer and more grounded. The plan also dovetailed with the formation of a representative, multidisciplinary, cross-department committee to establish clinical guidelines, policies, and procedures: 1 standard for practicing at DHMC. This approach has endured as one of the boldest and most positive changes for the collaborative practice. Privileges were brought in line with this change. Voluminous midwifery protocols were scrapped and a 1-page collaborative practice agreement took its place, to the delight of risk managers and compliance officers (Appendix 1, **Table 1**).

**Table 1**
**DHMC recommends constructing collaborative practice agreements and clinical practice guidelines as two distinct entities**

| Collaborative Practice Agreement | Clinical Practice Guidelines |
|---|---|
| One-page document that can be useful for a variety of purposes, such as in compliance and business venues | Collection of guidelines in which each addresses 1 *specific* clinical entity with goal of reducing unwarranted variation in practice |
| In agreement with ACNM and ACOG standards and positions | Evidence-based and in agreement with ACOG and ACNM standards and positions. Developed by a multi-disciplinary standing committee (OB MD, FP MD, CNM, RN, Ped, Anes) |
| Population you serve and where you practice | Set a standard of care that must be adhered to by all CNMs and MDs caring for the patient |
| Arrangement for consultation, referral, and comanagement | May contain "when to consult or refer" for specific clinical conditions; *or* this may be detailed in Clinical Privileges |
| Collaborating MD's responsibilities to uphold his/her part of this agreement | Allow for exceptions with clear documentation regarding rationale |
| CNM responsibilities to uphold his/her part of this agreement | Are easily accessed at all clinical sites |
| Must be updated on a schedule and maintenance must be assigned to a committee or to individual in a job description | Must be updated on a schedule and maintenance must be assigned to a committee or to individual in a job description. *Must be formatted to allow for easy and quick revision when new evidence emerges* |
| Outdated documents must be archived for use in insurance claims or lawsuits | Outdated documents must be archived for use in insurance claims or lawsuits |

*Abbreviations:* Anes, anesthesiology; Ped, pediatrics.

The close relationship with the MFM physicians changed the CNM's relationship with the generalist OB/GYNs who had previously been their closest colleagues. Combining the CNMs and APRNs into a single division created new professional bonds among them as well as opportunities for CNMs who wished to transition to new positions and work in the APRN role. Gynecology became the point of intersection for CNMs with generalist teams, reproductive endocrinology and infertility (REI), gynecologic oncology, and urogynecology.

The CNMs organized a continuing education program entitled CNMs and APRNs as Educators of Medical Students and Residents. Resident candidates heard about the collaborative practice from the MD and CNM viewpoints during their interview day and the CNM Director became involved in the resident selection process. The CNMs began a tradition of welcoming new residents with dinner and teaching sessions on the conduct of normal spontaneous vaginal delivery during their first week. For several years, first-year residents became Midwife-for-a-Month and they were fully integrated into the CNM service. When RRC resident duty hours and content requirements made this impossible to continue, every effort was made to address these learning needs during day-to-day contact on the inpatient unit. Presentations were made honoring each resident at graduation and Excellence in Teaching awards were given to CNMs and advanced registered nurse practitioners (ARNPs) from medical students and residents.

Dartmouth-Hitchcock MDs and CNMs realized that their collaborative practice was back on course when medical centers and professional associations regularly called for advice and mentorship. Once changes to the structure and functions of the practice were accomplished, a reevaluation of full-time equivalents, salary, workweek composition, and faculty rank began. These issues have presented ongoing challenges, as they have in many places, and permanent solutions have been hard to find.

## CHALLENGES AND SOLUTIONS: THIRD DECADE, 2003 TO THE PRESENT

The work of maintaining a collaborative practice demands stamina and resilience. Thanks to the hard work done by our predecessors and the commitment of our current department members, the collaborative nature of our practice is well entrenched in every aspect of our department as well as the DHMC organization. The MDs shared in the celebration and accolades when the CNMs were awarded the ACNM With Women, for a Lifetime Gold Commendation in 2005. However, challenges still remain and continued vigilance is required. In the increasingly complex health care delivery system, it is vital to continue to recognize the need for all concerned to find ways to contribute to the improvement of quality health care and participate in the education of various health care providers, while addressing cost containment. The Northern New England Perinatal Quality Improvement Network (NNEPQIN) has emerged as a resource and a forum for some of the difficult challenges the MDs and CNMs currently face. NNEPQIN was created in 2004 and grew out of the Vermont/New Hampshire VBAC project with a mission to improve perinatal care throughout northern New England. Membership is offered to hospital perinatal care teams, not individuals. NNEPQIN is a consensus-driven, horizontally structured, inclusive organization that provides cutting-edge educational programs, develops and shares clinical guidelines, and provides confidential case review for members. To this end, a provision was made for Vermont home birth midwives to join as a single team. Collaborative practice is at the heart of NNEPQIN's work and DHMC is an active team in its activities.

CNMs have become more involved in the business aspects of their practice, addressing financial dilemmas and adjusting practice patterns to address specific issues. Having representation on the Executive Leadership Team allows the CNMs to stay informed regarding pressures that the organization is experiencing and the solutions being discussed. Looking back from this third and current decade of collaborative practice, it would have been simpler for the MDs to move through the multiple stages in department development without the CNMs. The same may be observed when looking to the future. However, the conflict is that most of the MDs, generalists and subspecialists, recognize that the CNMs have distinguished themselves as clinicians and educators, some as novice researchers and published authors, and that the CNMs bring a dimension to the department that can be difficult to articulate. Our long history of developing ways to do things differently will serve us well as we continue to redesign care to optimize outcomes, meet the needs of the women in our care, and enhance our own professional development and job satisfaction.

### *Practice Model*

The practice model has been collaborative since its founding in 1983. Then, as now, CNMs carried their own panel of patients and had easy and frequent discussions with MDs for resolution of clinical issues. The MDs provided ready support and consultation during intrapartum care as needed. MDs concurrently sought opinions frequently from the CNMs. At first, the CNMs met weekly with an MD to present their caseload of patients, but this quickly changed to an agreement that the CNMs would speak with an MD if problems arose. A woman's choice of midwifery care was respected and she was transferred to MD care only when necessary and if all parties were in agreement. Secretaries, clinic assistants, and nurses who understood and respected both the MDs and CNMs were assets to the collaborative practice model from the beginning. Many of these essential features of collaborative practice have remained in place over the decades, but the easy informality of the early years has become more structured as the department has grown.

The physicians and CNMs continue to hold each other in high regard as people and as professionals, viewing differences as inevitable and potentially beneficial. Each has an awareness of the knowledge, skills, and perspectives of both professions, and both are recognized for making unique and important, but complementary, contributions to our common goal: excellent clinical outcomes and improved health status through sharing our knowledge and empowering the women in our care.

The Department of Obstetrics and Gynecology is currently composed of 6 divisions: CNMs and APRNs, General Obstetrics/Gynecology, REI, MFM, Urogynecology, and Gynecologic Oncology. Births all take place at DHMC, but all divisions provide outreach at additional sites in Vermont and New Hampshire. Providers include 8 CNMs, 6 APRNs, 25 physicians, and 16 residents.

A woman-centered model for deciding on care requires that women are involved in shaping their care. Shared medical appointments (SMAs) are strongly encouraged for all patients seeking obstetric care at DHMC, and most women attend at least 1 SMA for their intake visit. During the SMA, the same information is provided to all women seeking prenatal care at DHMC. Options for care (by the CNM or MD teams) as well as group visits are reviewed. These visits also include a discussion of prenatal screening options with one of the genetic counselors and a review of care content and important do's and don'ts for early pregnancy. Women who opt for care with the CNM team are then seen by members of that division. There are occasional transfers to the MFM team, but, even then, many high-risk patients are able to remain with the CNM team for most of their care and birth. The generalist OB/GYN teams include attending physicians, residents, and an APRN. Although we began with a model of offering separate group visits led by CNMs and MDs, we have since evolved to a model in which women seeking shared care are enrolled in the group that is appropriate for their gestational age, with the option to have either a physician or CNM attend the birth. This option would not be possible if our underlying philosophies of care were not similar, and if we were not equally convinced of the value of shared care. We also encourage women to explore their options, and support transfer from one team to another when requested. Over the years, the distribution of patients has remained about one-third CNMs, one-third generalist OB/GYNs, and one-third MFM and transports.

## LEADERSHIP

Collaborative practice takes more than good intentions. Supportive leadership and strong infrastructure are crucial to success. How decisions are made regarding patient care ultimately begins with the mission, vision, and goals identified by both the organization and, more specifically, the department. The Executive Leadership Team (ELT) of the Obstetrics/Gynecology Department consists of the Department Chair, Division Directors, Administrative Director, and Practice Manager. A retreat in 2008 reviewed the mission, vision, and goals and ensured that all divisions were united and working toward the common outcomes identified. Monthly meetings ensure that the communication is frequent and the absence of hierarchical approach lends itself to communication that is open, honest, strong, and shares power. Shared decision making starts at this level and ensures that the perspectives of various professions/disciplines are taken into consideration.

Shared responsibility implies that all involved professions cooperate in the collaborative process and have accountability for the outcome. In the current litigious environment, CNMs and MDs must articulate who has the duty of care in each situation, as well as when they share it or transfer it. Collaborative practice works when everyone practices to the full extent, and not beyond their training and licensure. Midwives who push the scope of practice boundaries and physicians who deflect difficult decision making and are reluctant to perform technical procedures are not a good match for collaborative practice. When asked by ACOG colleagues in 2010 whether the MDs should supervise CNMs, Emily Baker, MD, Director of Maternal-Fetal Medicine, responded that "As a result of their education and training, obstetrician-gynecologists take the unique responsibility for overseeing the response to obstetric emergencies and for managing obstetric emergencies which require surgical intervention. They also take the responsibility for immediate availability for consultation to other members of the team. They may be called on to take a leadership role or share in a leadership role with another team member. The contributions of each team member are valued and important to the quality of patient outcomes."

Over the years, a variety of issues have been brought to the ELT. These issues include hiring/recruitment processes based on key characteristics; enlightened financial reporting and analysis structure, including profit and loss reporting, productivity measures, and transparency; disciplinary procedures and performance appraisals; quality assurance (QA) and disciplinary processes in which all providers are held equally accountable to a high level of standards; and decisions regarding models of care at clinical outreach sites.

In making decisions about staffing and systems at outreach sites, the ELT members discussed the mandate to keep the department on a productive and profitable course and simultaneously they brought forward practical, clinical, service-oriented considerations. They made a plan in which the CNMs provide the prenatal care at outreach sites. Generalist OB/GYNs do limited outreach sessions and focus on complex and surgical gynecology at these sites. Subspecialist MDs are carefully scheduled to maximize their effectiveness and ease referrals. The ELT worked creatively, cooperatively, and in concert with the Dartmouth-Hitchcock vision: Achieve the healthiest population possible, leading the transformation of health care in our region and setting the standard for our nation.

## STATE, REGULATORY, AND CREDENTIALING ISSUES

New Hampshire legislation and regulations have been conducive to the formation of collaborative practices between CNMs and physicians. Representatives of the Dartmouth-Hitchcock organization and members of the Department of Obstetrics and Gynecology have had a strong voice in resolving legislative and regulatory issues as they evolved over time.

CNMs in New Hampshire are regulated by the Board of Nursing, under the terms of the Nurse Practice Act, and are licensed as APRNs. They must possess a current RN license and a graduate degree earned in an accredited APRN education program (there are separate provisions for those who graduated before 2004) and hold current certification by a board-recognized certifying body in the specialty for which the APRN was educated. Scope of practice is defined as performing acts of advanced assessment, diagnosing, prescribing, selecting, administering, and providing therapeutic measures and treatment regimes; and obtaining consultation, planning, implementing collaborative management, referral, or transferring the care of the client as appropriate. The statute specifies that APRNs may perform other functions for which they are educationally and experientially prepared and are consistent with standards established by national credentialing and certifications bodies. APRNs have plenary authority to possess, compound, prescribe, administer, and dispense and distribute to clients controlled and noncontrolled drugs within the scope of the APRN's practice. For many years, prescriptive authority was granted via an official formulary established by The Joint Health Council, which consisted of MDs, pharmacists, and APRNs. The Joint Health Council was legislatively repealed on July 1, 2009.[1] CNMs may sign birth certificates. Since 1985, New Hampshire has mandated fee-for-service reimbursement for all APRNs, including CNMs, by all insurance companies. The state Medicaid program reimburses CNMs at 100% of physician fee levels.[2]

No statutory or regulatory provision requires hospitals to provide access by CNMs to clinical or admitting privileges or prohibits discrimination against them in granting such privileges. At DHMC, until 1992, the obstetrician/gynecologists, CNMs, and ARNPs were members of the Department of Maternal and Child Health and the Section of Gynecology in the Department of Surgery. Credentialing and privileging responsibilities devolved to the Chair (a pediatrician) and to the Section Chief (an obstetrician/gynecologist.) Original credentialing involved minimal documentation of training, licensure, board status, and degrees. The requirements for state licensure for CNMs and nurse practitioners for the state became more specific and rigorous over time and were always prerequisites for practice at our medical center. The specificity and rigorousness of the privileging documents increased over time. In the 1980s, the nurse-midwifery privileges were primarily for care of only low-risk women. Privileges for early nurse practitioners were devoid of specificity other than a few minor surgical procedures. During this era, a physician had privileges for every possible condition and treatment at the level of a specialist or subspecialist as warranted by level of training.

In 1995, DHMC formed a Task Force on Credentialing and Privileging for Advanced Practice Nurses and asked the Director of the Nurse-Midwifery Service to serve as Cochair. The work of this group resulted in the CNMs becoming Active Professional Staff members appointed and reappointed through the Credentials Committee. A CNM was invited to serve on the DHMC Credentials Committee to assist in the transition to credentialing nonphysician providers across the organization, which coincided with the creation of the Department of Obstetrics and Gynecology.

Three years later, the Department of Obstetrics and Gynecology convened a work group to revise obstetric privileging and credentialing. The members comprised the Director, Division of Midwives and Nurse Practitioners; Director, Division of Maternal-Fetal Medicine; a generalist obstetrician; Clinical Chief, Department of Community and Family Medicine at the medical center; and 2 community-based family physicians. The qualifications for eligibility for application for privileges were specified, including training, board certification, recent patient care volumes, continuing medical education, and peer evaluation. Three categories of care were established: primary-care obstetrics with certified nurse-midwives and family physicians, specialty-care obstetrics with generalist obstetrician-gynecologists, and subspecialty-care obstetrics with MFM physicians. A document was crafted that delineated responsibilities to the patients and responsibilities across provider groups. Participation in continuing medical education, departmental conferences, and institutional clinical practice workgroups became an expectation for all providers. Regardless of level of training or experience, the document specified that all new providers must have their first 6 births proctored by a currently privileged CNM or MD who is not necessarily from that person's practice group. A privilege document was developed that outlined which conditions could be managed independently, which needed consultation, and which needed referral to consultants. This process provided clarity on roles and responsibilities of all providers and an understanding of the interdependence of disciplines, which has also proved valuable in assigning responsibilities for resident education and training: CNMs teach those functions and procedures that they themselves have privileges to perform.

### *Practice Outcomes*

From the beginning, the CNMs collected data to document their outcomes. Analysis of their data was regularly published in departmental reports and presented at Grand Rounds. As departmental data collection evolved, there was a period of time in which CNM and MD outcomes were presented in a competitive way. When it was recognized that this could erode team relationships and function, the CNMs revised the language with which their practice information and outcomes were presented.

In 2003, OBNet, a Web-based delivery registry jointly developed by DHMC and Fletcher Allen Health Care, was introduced. It allows the generation of hospital-specific reports with patient-identified clinical data for internal QA efforts and deidentified reports used in regional quality improvement efforts and benchmarking. We are able to review outcomes by individual providers or groups of providers. Review of outcomes is a regular part of department meetings, and OBNet data are the primary source for information on the DHMC Public Reporting Web site's Pregnancy Care page (http://patients.dartmouth-hitchcock.org/quality/quality_report/PC).[3] Prompted by a query from a visitor to the Web site about why MD and CNM results were not presented separately, because they must be different, we compared outcomes for the

CNM and generalist teams. There were identical rates of cesarean sections, primary cesarean sections, episiotomy, and operative vaginal delivery. DHMC also remains a tertiary care center with an epidural rate of about 45%; this is now proving to be an attractor for students and residents who have not had the opportunity to see, let alone learn, to manage, an unmedicated birth. OBNet also allows us to investigate a specific provider's practice, enhancing our department's ability to document questionable clinical issues/practices and support patient-safety initiatives. In our QA and disciplinary processes, standards are high and nurse-midwives and physicians are held to them.

Since 2007, as a result of gathering data through OBNet, the CNM service has participated in the ACNM benchmarking program. Using quality metrics, the program compares data for participating midwifery practices. It compares like-sized practices and reports on their outcomes to "improve and maintain the quality of midwifery care provided to women and children by promoting member awareness of "best practices." (http://www.midwife.org/ACNM/files/ccLibraryFiles/Filename/000000000530/Sample_Benchmarking_Survey.pdf).[4]

The Dartmouth-Hitchcock organization conducted a review of cases reported to the Claims Manager between 1995 and 2010. Findings were used to inform QA, quality improvement, and patient-safety work. More than 90% of the cases were reported within days of the event by the RN, CNM, or MD who rendered the care. The organizational culture favors a low threshold for reporting. This series of cases provided another view into the collaborative practice. This study was conducted by a CNM and generalist OB/GYN with specialty consultants as needed. Over the 15-year study period, there were a few cases involving the CNMs and settlement amounts were minimal by industry standards. The cases for which reserves were set aside involved intrapartum management and were characterized by CNMs and MDs working closely during the care. The reviewers noted that a robust organization-wide risk management and claims management program was in place during the study period. Specific to collaborative practice, clinical guidelines that are followed by RNs, CNMs, and MDs and have all parties insured by the same captive were factors in favorable claims outcomes. In addition, CNMs and MDs emerged from claims and suits as trusted colleagues despite the traumatic nature of litigation. Although claims data review does not afford the same rigor as other measurement methods, the professional liability history of this collaborative practice has provided insight into the quality of the clinical practice and an alternative way to look at the cost-effectiveness of the model.

### *Interdisciplinary Education and Training*

Interprofessional education (IPE) occurs when "two or more professions learn with, from, and about each other" (Center for the Advancement of Interprofessional Education).[5] Although recently recognized by the World Health Organization as a "necessary component of every health professional's education,"[6] interprofessional education has been a prominent feature for learners at DHMC from the beginning. Obstetricians and nurse-midwives have shared training sessions on normal birth, and these have been, and still are, as important as those on managing emergencies. The DHMC CNMs have always participated in the teaching of medical students. This participation was particularly effective when we recruited women volunteers as teaching assistants for breast and pelvic examination, with CNMs doing much of the mentoring and modeling of behavior. A major improvement was the joint approach to the objective structured clinical examination. The CNMs advocated inclusion of skills such as teaching women how to take birth control pills, nutrition assessment and counseling, and conducting a postpartum visit, and these were added to the list of skills assessed along with the surgical skills. There have existed many barriers to interprofessional education, but the major one has been the historical hierarchy in the health care setting that identified physicians as the most powerful professionals.[7] This was not the case at DHMC. “Our practice has prepared many residents to enter practices where they are in a collaborative arrangement with CNMs which has been a great help in community hospitals that have difficulty recruiting good maternity providers” (Chair Emeritus, Department of Obstetrics and Gynecology, Barry D. Smith, MD, personal communication, 2010).

The Accreditation Council on Graduate Medical Education currently requires that residents learn to work in interdisciplinary teams. “Our residents have a genuine understanding of what it means to be partners with CNMs,” observes Tina Foster MD, an OB/GYN who directs a leadership program at The Dartmouth Institute for Health Policy and Clinical Practice. A recent trend noted in interviews with applicants for residency is candidates who are specifically looking for training programs in which CNMs are an integral part of the practice and in which the skills of working with CNMs can be developed. The CNMs, realizing that they are an aging workforce, have welcomed younger colleagues into the practice when others have moved out of the area or to work as APRNs with other divisions within the department. Watching the younger CNMs form relationships with residents and staff MDs closer to their age provides hope for the future of the collaborative practice.

The dedication to interprofessional education continues to be seen at every level within the department and organization. The Director for the Division of APRNs and CNMs is a member of both the Resident Education Committee and Student Education Committee, promoting the role of APRNs and CNMs in medical and residency education. She also continues to participate in the interview and selection process for incoming residents. Prospective residents are already aware that collaborative practice is a concept that is embraced by both leadership and clinicians. The APRNs and CNMs continue to provide didactic sessions to medical students and residents as well as mentoring sessions both in the outpatient and inpatient settings.

A key component of maintaining collaboration is to participate jointly in needs assessments for change in practice. Department-sponsored morbidity and mortality conferences, monthly obstetric case conferences, and weekly Grand Rounds provide these opportunities. The first 2 conferences in particular lend themselves to audience participation in the discussion and public demonstration of respect for each other’s opinions. Ongoing drills of obstetric emergencies promote team training. Physicians and CNMs all take part in simulations both in-situ and in the DHMC Patient Safety and Training Center, which provides high-fidelity simulation equipment and video-enhanced debriefing.

## SUMMARY

Barbara Fildes CNM, third CNM Director, observed that “The CNMs and MDs at Dartmouth-Hitchcock, like their colleagues everywhere, work within a context filled with family triumph and heartbreak, colleagues arriving and leaving, illness and recovery, victory and disaster both close to home and far away. In a strong collaborative practice, these experiences are always considered and respected. They serve as points of poignant intersection among staff but they are neither the basis nor the focus of the practice. These shared experiences create bonds but do not guarantee the survival of collaborative practice.” Mickey Cordell CNM, the current Director, emphasizes that "events and experiences can greatly affect day-to-day operations of the department but they do not disrupt our focus on the mission, vision, and goals. Maintaining this focus during times of celebration or times of trauma is the job of CNM and MD clinical leaders."

A checklist of essential elements for sustainable collaborative practice is presented at the end of this article (Appendix 2). As we conclude our reflections, it is vital to point out that collaborative practice is about more than just a practice model or a set of items that, once checked off, will guarantee success. We could not tell this story without invoking the names and memories of the courageous individuals who took the bold first steps, or revisiting the memories of those who struggled in the adolescent years of our practice, or those who lead us now. The success of our collaboration is linked to the focus and dedication of all our clinicians to providing the best care possible to the women in our care. Do we get it right 100% of the time? No, but we know how to look honestly at where we could do better and tackle those areas with the same enthusiasm as we bring to designing a new program or helping a new life enter the world. Our confidence in each other, the trust that we display, and the respect for each others' ways of doing things are what enable us to have the difficult conversations that are needed for successful collaborative practice. It is the collective ability to value each other and what we bring to the whole that has helped us to weave (and to continue weaving) our individual threads into a rich tapestry of practice around the warp of our shared aims and vision for what women's health care can be. We finished this writing process with a renewed sense of gratitude for our predecessors, our current colleagues, our community of practice in both medicine and midwifery, and great hopes for the future that our current trainees will build.

Richard Reindollar, MD, Chair, Department of Obstetrics and Gynecology, describes our program: "The practice of obstetrics at Dartmouth has evolved over 30 years into a uniquely collaborative pattern of care. On the surface it looks like 3 separate practices nearly equally divided: MFM, general obstetrics, and nurse-midwifery. However, the whole is truly bigger than the sum of the parts, as individual perspectives of care have become a shared philosophy."

## REFERENCES

1. Practice/Licensure - N.H. Rev. Stat. Ann. Chapter 326-B: §§ 11,18 (2005).
2. Birth Certificates - N.H. Rev. Stat. Ann. Chapter 5-C: §§ 19-40, 74–89 (2005).
3. Dartmouth-Hitchcock Medical Center. Practice outcomes-pregnancy performance results. Available at: http://patients.dartmouth-hitchcock.org/quality/quality_report/PC. Accessed January 24, 2012.
4. American College of Nurse-Midwives (ACNM) benchmarking program. sample benchmarking survey. 2012. Available at: http://www.midwife.org/ACNM/files/ccLibraryFiles/Filename/000000000530/Sample_Benchmarking_Survey.pdf. Accessed January 24, 2012.
5. Rodger S, Hoffman S, World Health Organization Study Group on Interprofessional Education and Collaborative Practice. Where in the world is interprofessional education? A global environmental scan. J Interprof Care 2010;24(5):479–91.
6. Yan J, Gilbert J, Hoffman SJ. World Health Organization Study Group on Interprofessional Education and Collaborative Practice. J Interprof Care 2007;22:588–9.
7. Freshman B, Rubino L, Chassiakos Y. Collaboration across the disciplines in health care. Sudbury (MA): Jones and Barlett; 2010.

## APPENDIX 1: COLLABORATIVE PRACTICE AGREEMENT BETWEEN PHYSICIANS, CERTIFIED NURSE-MIDWIVES, AND ADVANCED REGISTERED NURSE PRACTITIONERS AT DHMC

**COLLABORATIVE PRACTICE AGREEMENT**
**BETWEEN PHYSICIANS, CERTIFIED NURSE-MIDWIVES,**
**and ADVANCED REGISTERED NURSE PRACTITIONERS**
**AT DARTMOUTH-HITCHCOCK MEDICAL CENTER**
**Department of Obstetrics and Gynecology**

The Department of Obstetrics and Gynecology, Dartmouth Hitchcock Medical Center, Lebanon NH, is a collaborative practice consisting of physicians , certified nurse-midwives (CNMs), and advanced practice registered nurses (APRNs) serving women with obstetrical, gynecological, and general health needs.

CNMs/ARNPs practice at Dartmouth-Hitchcock Clinic sites in New Hampshire and Vermont and at Mary Hitchcock Memorial Hospital in Lebanon, NH.

CNMs/APRNs care for a variety of female patients in collaboration with department physicians as members of the following clinical teams:

- Nurse-Midwifery Service
- ambulatory Generalist Ob/Gyn
- Gynecologic Oncology
- Reproductive Endocrinology and Infertility
- Urogynecology

The physicians in the Department of Obstetrics and Gynecology serve as collaborating physicians for the CNMs/APRNs under the direction of the Chair. Generalist obstetrician-gynecologists and subspecialist physicians in Maternal-Fetal Medicine, Gynecologic Oncology, Urogynecology, and Reproductive Endocrinology & Infertility are available and accessible twenty-four hours per day for consultation and referral. There is an obstetrician-gynecologist on site at the Dartmouth-Hitchcock Medical Center, Lebanon NH at all times.

CNMs/APRNs complete a credentialing and privileging process through the DHMC Office of Clinical Affairs and the DHMC Credentials Committee. CNMs/APRNs function as Active Clinical Staff in accordance with:

- State law
- Professional Staff Bylaws and Rules and Regulations
- DHMC and departmental policies and practice guidelines
- job description
- individual privileges in obstetrics and gynecology
- standards established by the individual's professional and certifying organization(s)
- DHMC and department mission, vision, and goals statements
- DHMC Code of Ethical Conduct

CNMs/APRNs participate in the following activities:

- structured orientation upon hire
- scheduled and unscheduled meetings with consulting physicians and peers
- annual performance appraisal
- multi-disciplinary committees addressing clinical care issues
- departmental OB Morbidity and Mortality Review, departmental Gyn Morbidity and Mortality Review,
- Tumor Board, Journal Club, Ethics Conference, Ob/Gyn Grand Rounds
- departmental Quality Assurance, Clinical Quality Improvement , and Patient Safety activities
- other projects and committees initiated by the DHMC, the department, or the Division.

| ______________________ | ______________________ |
|---|---|
| Chair<br>Department, Obstetrics & Gynecology | Director<br>Division, Nurse-Midwives and Nurse Practitioners |

## APPENDIX 2: CHECKLIST: ESSENTIAL ELEMENTS FOR SUSTAINABLE COLLABORATIVE CNM/MD PRACTICE

*Choose partners wisely.* You cannot collaborate with someone who does not want to collaborate with you.

- ☐ Team involved in MD and CNM hiring
- ☐ MDs involved in midwifery student clinical placement
- ☐ CNMs involved in residency selection
- ☐ Individuals are hired who will hold each other in high regard as people and professionals, while viewing their differences as inevitable and potentially beneficial

*Build and maintain strong infrastructure.* Collaborative practice takes more than good intentions.

- ☐ CNM and MD leaders have job descriptions, accountability, compensation, and place on organizational chart
- ☐ CNMs and MDs have job descriptions
- ☐ CNMs and MDs have clearly articulated salary and benefits
- ☐ Recruitment tools with key characteristics are used for each search
- ☐ Organization's by-laws support CNM/MD collaboration
- ☐ Faculty appointments are made
- ☐ Credentialing and privileging process is in place
- ☐ Billing and coding maximizes revenue
- ☐ Financial analysis and reporting captures CNM and MD overlapping and distinct contributions
- ☐ Professional liability insurance provided by same entity
- ☐ Collaborative Practice Agreement is separate from Clinical Practice Guidelines
- ☐ Clinical Practice Guidelines are developed by multi-disciplinary committee(s)
- ☐ QA indicators are tied to Clinical Guidelines
- ☐ Chain of Communication policy is clear and effective
- ☐ Due process and disciplinary procedures are in place
- ☐ Succession planning is on-going
- ☐ Infrastructure in compliance with federal and state legislation and regulations

*Make accountability for clinical outcomes the core requirement for CNMs and MDs.* A collaborative practice works best when CNM and MD efforts remain directed toward excellent clinical outcomes and improved health status for women in their community.

- ☐ Measures are in place, understood, and utilized by CNMs and MDs.
- ☐ CNM and MD leaders assure that CNMs and MDs practice to the full extent of their training and licensure, and not beyond.
- ☐ CNM and MD leaders set standards high and hold everyone to them.
- ☐ CNM and MD leaders articulate that while some clinical outcomes can be attributed to either CNMs or MDs, it is the aggregate outcomes that are most important

*Teach and support each other's young and inexperienced.* They become your pool of potential colleagues in a few years. Use your limited resources wisely and determine what kind of teaching fits your practice.

- ☐ EMS personnel, childbirth educators, and doulas
- ☐ Nurses
- ☐ Nurse practitioners
- ☐ Medical students
- ☐ Midwifery students
- ☐ Residents in pediatrics, anesthesia, family practice, and others
- ☐ Ob/Gyn Residents
- ☐ Recently trained or inexperienced CNMs and MDs
- ☐ CNMs and MDs needing remediation

*Connect practice with those addressing similar challenges.* Few clinicians have the time and resources to devote to issues that have been thoroughly researched and addressed by peers and/or experts.

- ☐ CNMs and MDs participate in key organizational initiatives and committees
- ☐ CNMs and MDs participate in ACNM, ACOG, regional quality initiatives and other groups with shared mission
- ☐ This contribution is supported in some way by the practice as a whole

*Abbreviation:* EMS, emergency medical system.

# Collaborative Practice Model

## Madigan Army Medical Center

Peter E. Nielsen, MD[a], Michelle Munroe, CNM[b], Lisa Foglia, MD[c], Roxanne I. Piecek, CNM[d], Mary Paul Backman, CNM[e], Rebecca Cypher, MSN, PNNP[e], Denise C. Smith, CNM[f,*]

**KEYWORDS**

• Collaboration between midwives and obstetricians • Graduate medical education
• Delivery of healthcare • Military medicine

**KEY POINTS**

- This article outlines the structure and processes for establishing a collaborative midwife-physician practice in a military academic medical center.
- Preliminary data suggests a reduction in primary c-section rates after implementation of the new practice model, though further investigation is needed to confirm this finding.
- Integration of midwifery faculty into resident education has been beneficial to patients, residents and staff.

The United States spends more than double per capita on health care compared with other industrialized nations, but ranks far below many developed countries in key perinatal outcomes, including maternal mortality, neonatal mortality rates, and cesarean section rates.[1] Reasons for these disparate outcomes are complex and some factors are beyond medical control. However, recent reports, including the Institute of Medicine's (IOM) "Crossing the Quality Chasm" (2001),[2] the Milbank Report "Evidenced-Based Maternity Care: What It Is and What it Can Achieve" (2008),[3] and the recent "2020 Vision for High-Value, High-Quality Maternity Care System,"[4] present as part of the solution to improve collaboration among different services and providers, including an increase in the use of midwifery care in the United States.

[a] Western Regional Medical Command, BLDG 2006, Liggett Ave., Joint Base Lewis McChord, WA 98433, USA; [b] Kenner Army Health Clinic, 700 24th Street, Fort Lee, VA 23801, USA; [c] OB/GYN Residency Program, Madigan Army Medical Center, 9040 A. Fitzsimmons Drive, Tacoma, WA 98431, USA; [d] Nurse-Midwifery Service, Madigan Army Medical Center, 9040 A. Fitzsimmons Drive, Tacoma, WA 98431, USA; [e] Madigan Army Medical Center, 9040 A. Fitzsimmons Drive, Tacoma, WA 98431, USA; [f] College of Nursing, University of Colorado, Mail Stop C28813120, East 19th Avenue, Aurora, CO 80045, USA
* Corresponding author. 912 Kadel Court, Geneseo, IL 61254.
*E-mail address:* denise.smith@ucdenver.edu

Obstet Gynecol Clin N Am 39 (2012) 399–410
http://dx.doi.org/10.1016/j.ogc.2012.05.008 **obgyn.theclinics.com**
0889-8545/12/$ – see front matter 

The IOM identified 6 aims for overall improvement in the quality of care, which includes care that is safe, effective, timely, efficient, equitable, and patient-centered and is based on the best available evidence. Evidence suggests that procedure-intense care leads to higher costs and poor patient outcomes.[3] It is unclear what role the use of such practices as continuous fetal monitoring, labor induction, epidural anesthesia, elective primary cesarean section, and repeat cesarean delivery play with respect to costs and patient outcomes.[3] However, the evidence supports that noninvasive practices, such as smoking cessation programs, group model prenatal care, continuous labor support, nonsupine positions for birth, and external cephalic versions, can improve perinatal outcomes. Consequently, the IOM has recommended that changes in the maternity care system are a priority.[5] A potential solution to reforming maternity care and promoting the use of noninvasive, evidenced-based practices is to use a maternity care delivery model that brings together midwives and obstetricians in a collaborative practice. The purpose of this article was to describe a successful collaborative practice model between physicians and midwives in a military medical center and outline how this care delivery model can provide quality obstetric care.

## MADIGAN ARMY MEDICAL CENTER, DEPARTMENT OF OBSTETRICS AND GYNECOLOGY

Madigan Army Medical Center (MAMC) is a tertiary care center serving active duty, family members, and military retirees in the Pacific Northwest with an enrolled population of approximately 110,000 and a referral population of more than 200,000. The Department of Obstetrics and Gynecology has a robust graduate medical education program including a residency program and maternal-fetal medicine fellowship. Annual volume is approximately 2400 births and includes a diverse population.

Since 2002, midwives have been part of the MAMC staff. At its inception, 2 full-time active-duty military certified nurse midwives (CNM) provided antenatal care with occasional intrapartum care. The midwives conducted antepartum, postpartum, and well-woman visits in the clinic 4 days a week and staffed the labor and delivery unit 1 day per week to accommodate resident education. This system was displeasing for many of the patients, as well as the residents and staff physicians, for a variety of reasons. Midwives did not feel that they were viewed as a valuable or integral member of the team. Patients often requested a midwife to attend their birth, which was not usually possible. Last, there was limited professional interaction between the CNM staff and resident physicians.

The National Defense Authorization Act of 2002[6] included a provision that pregnant TRICARE beneficiaries were allowed to seek prenatal care in civilian facilities without out-of-pocket expense. Because our facility could not accommodate patients' request for midwifery-specific care, an increasing number of MAMC patients requested obstetric care by civilian midwives.

In 2003, the Accreditation Council for Graduate Medical Education (ACGME) instituted new standards for the maximum number of weekly duty hours for residents in their accredited programs.[7] In addition to the limit in duty hours, the ACGME recommended other changes to the resident duty hours that had a significant impact on an institution's ability to maintain a continuous physician presence in the hospital. Decreasing the number of resident hours meant that there would be fewer residents covering inpatient services. Residents and staff were challenged to staff labor and delivery in compliance with these new ACGME work-hour guidelines, with the concern that additional work-hour restrictions would evolve over time. Indeed, work-hour restrictions, now to include limitation of intern work hours to a maximum of 16 hours per day, effectively eliminated the traditional 24-hour call for residents in postgraduate year 1 (PGY-1) as of the 2011–2012 academic year.

Based on these circumstances and the desire to improve the woman's intrapartum experience, MAMC formed a midwifery service within the organizational structure of the Department of Obstetrics and Gynecology. The purpose of this article is to describe this collaborative practice.

## COLLABORATIVE PRACTICE MODEL

Collaboration takes place between 2 individuals or among groups of people that cover a variety of practices. For the purposes of this article, collaboration is defined in terms of the relationship between midwives and physicians who are obstetric providers. Collaboration can be defined as the successful coordination of activities between 2 individuals or groups working toward a shared goal, where each entity has a role in the planning, decision making, problem solving, and responsibility of the overall task.[8] Successful collaboration with obstetricians is crucial to midwifery practice, particularly with regard to the midwife's scope of practice. Midwifery care is focused on the care of healthy women, whereas advanced obstetric care, provided by obstetricians and maternal-fetal medicine subspecialists, is essential for the care of women with high-risk pregnancies and those women who develop complications during pregnancy. The relationship between the midwife and physician scope of practice and management of care is depicted in **Fig. 1**. The American College of Nurse-Midwives and the American College of Obstetricians and Gynecologists (ACOG) have acknowledged the importance of this collaborative relationship in a joint statement.[9] The collaborative practice at MAMC was designed with consideration of scope of practice, concerns for enhancing resident education, and a desire to improve prenatal care options for patients and thus increase patient satisfaction.

Collaboration and teamwork are integral to successfully accomplishing complicated tasks. The 2003 IOM report recommends that institutions engaged in clinical education develop and work in interdisciplinary teams.[10] MAMC has been a leader in team training in medicine, which led to the first-ever randomized clinical trial of medical team training in 2003.[11] This model is predicated on collaboration of all team members and includes key components: team leadership, situation monitoring, mutual support, and communication.[11–13]

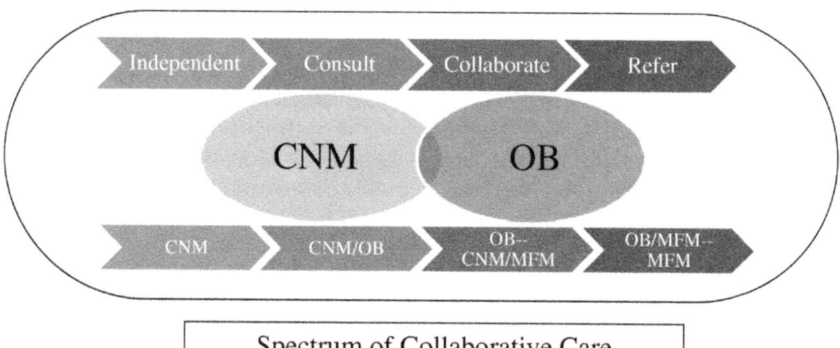


**Fig. 1.** Scope of practice and management of care between physicians and midwives.

Therefore, in 2006, the department developed a strategic plan to develop a collaborative model, with 3 goals:

1. Provide a 24/7 midwifery service. This required hiring additional midwives to ensure the ability to provide antepartum outpatient service and labor and delivery, with the ability to guarantee CNM presence at the delivery of patients empaneled to the CNM service.
2. Fully integrate the midwifery service into resident education. CNMs were incorporated into inpatient supervision of interns managing normal labor and delivery triage and uncomplicated deliveries, participation in resident and medical student didactic teaching, and attendance at perinatal morbidity and mortality conferences. In addition, CNM attendance was incorporated into our semiannual faculty meetings. To further enhance the role of the CNMs in collaborative teamwork, the CNM labor and delivery shift changes were adjusted to coincide with reporting of the medical, nursing, and anesthesia teams at 0700 and 1900. Midwives were expected to discuss evidence-based clinical practice and instruct medical students, off-service residents, and categorical interns in the midwifery model of care.
3. Ensure that all pregnant TRICARE beneficiaries were provided the opportunity to enroll in dedicated midwifery services in our military treatment facility. This allowed us to satisfy the patient's desire for the midwifery model of care while reducing health care costs to our institution by decreasing referrals to civilian hospitals for midwifery care. In addition, CNM patients typically desire fewer interventions, thus decreasing procedurally based health care costs. At Madigan, midwife patients were the first patients to ambulate during labor, use intermittent monitoring protocols, birthing balls, and hydrotherapy for pain management.

The process of developing a 24/7 CNM service began in January 2007 with 3 CNMs, who provided 24/7 coverage of midwifery patients. At that time, 20 patients per month were in the dedicated CNM panel. They were self-selected, low risk, and desired minimal-intervention midwifery care. After 6 months and many earned hours of compensatory time and overtime, the justification to hire additional midwifery staff was completed and approved by the hospital board. As of 2010, the service has 7 full-time CNMs (1 active duty and 6 civilians) and 1 part-time CNM providing 24/7, in-house coverage of labor and delivery, along with outpatient antepartum care. Currently, the panel accommodates 45 patients per month. These patients all receive continuity care with the CNM service and CNM intrapartum care. A single maternal–fetal medicine subspecialist provides consultation to the service for antepartum care and the labor and delivery unit physician staff provides intrapartum consultation as needed.

While on the labor and delivery unit, the CNMs are actively involved in intern and medical student education. They participate in supervision of labor and delivery triage and deliveries of obstetric service patients, when participation does not compromise their commitment to the empaneled CNM patients. Nurse-midwifery students are also part of this education program, which we believe enhances CNM student/resident physician relationships and sets the groundwork for favorable future collaborative relations.

### *Essential Elements of Collaborative Practice*

There are different theoretical bases for characterizing collaborative models of care. Systems theory, organizational theory, and group dynamics models have all been used to describe the elements of successful practice,[14] and most models describe elements such as attitudes of trust, congruence of philosophy, effective communication, organized processes, appreciation of differences, competence, and shared responsibility.[15–17] Miller[15] describes the different levels of collaboration: dysfunctional, just functional, disorganized but philosophically congruent, organized but philosophically incongruent, and synergistic supercollaboration (**Fig. 2**). Dysfunctional organizations have neither a common philosophy nor an organized structure, resulting in harm to the patient or the provider. Just functional organizations are similar to the dysfunctional, except that no harm occurs. Disorganized, but philosophically congruent and the organized, but philosophically incongruent groups lack one characteristic or the other. These practices tended to function adequately, but lack the characteristics to flourish. A synergistic practice creates a positive cycle of working together, increasing trust and patient satisfaction, which perpetuates and builds the confidence of the team over time. This physician/CNM relationship is depicted in **Fig. 2**. The basis of this working relationship is a firm belief in the value of the physician-midwife collaboration, and is what we believe our practice at MAMC represents.

Communication could be considered as the most critical element in collaboration and teamwork. Communication is ideally open and honest, regular, bi-directional, accurate, clear, concise, and systematic.[13,14,17] Communication can be formal or informal.[14] Formal communication includes morning report, board checkouts, team meetings, patient handoffs, resident faculty meetings, risk management activities, and medical record documentation. It is structured, follows predictable patterns, and is a means of sharing information. Informal communication is anything other than structured communication.[14] Informal methods of communication are more common and likely as important to the success of a team as formal methods.

## *Outcomes in Successful Collaborative Practice*

### *Patient and provider satisfaction*

Patient satisfaction surveys have revealed positive results both quantitatively and anecdotally. MAMC midwives consistently have a 90% or higher satisfaction rating

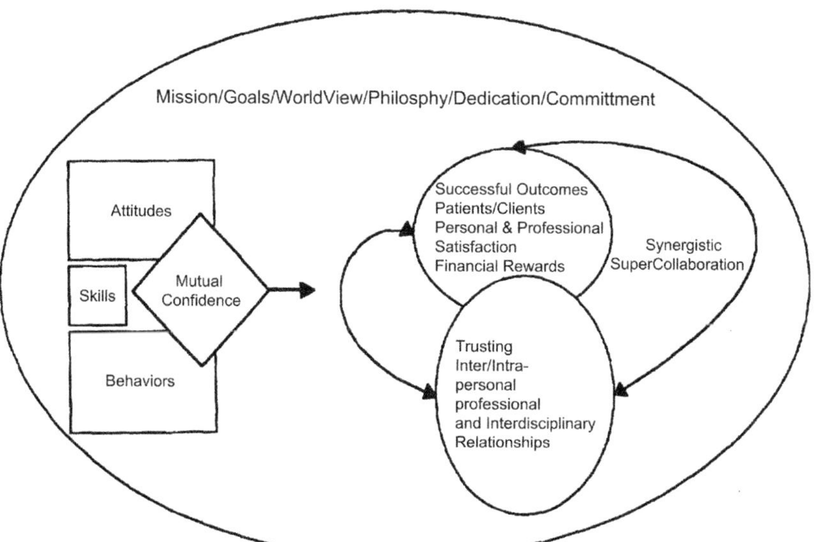


**Fig. 2.** Miller Model of Midwife Physician Collaboration. (*From* Miller S. Midwives' and physicians' experience in collaborative practice: a qualitative study. Womens Health Issues 1997;7(5):301–8; with permission.)

in survey data. Resident supervision by CNMs on labor and delivery has increased. During 2007, 130 resident-attended births were supervised by CNMs; by 2010, this increased to 178 births. **Tables 1–3** demonstrate the rates of analgesia, anesthesia, interventions, and birth outcomes. The following quote demonstrates how this collaboration is viewed by a woman enrolled in group prenatal care.

> *"I wasn't sure what to expect when they told us our group would be co-facilitated by a midwife and an obstetrician. I thought, are they going to argue all the time? When I saw group after group that they treated each other with respect and laughed together, it made me know they had the same goals even though they approached them with different educations." (Patient in group prenatal care where CNM was mentor to a second-year obstetrician/gynecologist resident [OB/GYN R2])*
>
> *"The obstetrician introduced the midwife as his colleague...like he meant it! After I saw him ask her opinion several times, I realized he DID mean it! That's cool. (Patient response on a postpartum survey, referring to her care while in labor.)*
>
> *"I found that midwives teach you without a lecture. Every day we worked together, I left knowing I had been taught new information, but in a manner that would stick. No one ever approached the discussion of contraception like the midwife I worked with. I never knew you could be so direct; so honest and so non-offensive all in the same sentence. I hope I will be able to do it that way, too. (R2 OB/GYN evaluation comment regarding working with a CNM as his staff.)*

***Vaginal birth after cesarean and trials of labor after cesarean section (TOLAC)***

Our institution meets all criteria outlined by ACOG[18] to offer trial of labor after cesarean section. In 2007, the CNM service deliveries accounted for 8% of the successful vaginal births after cesarean (VBACs) in our department. By 2010, this increased to 21% of the department's successful VBACs. The collaborative practice atmosphere creates an environment that is fully supportive of CNM providers managing patients undergoing VBAC attempt, and all eligible candidates are encouraged to attempt this route of delivery.

***Initiation of evidence-based practices***

Group prenatal care was initiated at Madigan in 2006 by one midwife. By December 2010, all CNMs were participating in group prenatal care. After successfully establishing the program among the CNM staff, several staff and resident physicians have completed the training and are involved in group prenatal care. For PGY-1/2 residents, group prenatal care provides an effective means to satisfy direct supervision requirements, to train and assess residents in all 6 of the ACGME core competencies, and to instruct trainees in the care of uncomplicated obstetric patients.

Continuous labor support is difficult in our setting for both the OB service and the CNM service because of the consistently high volume of patients admitted to labor and delivery. CNMs are usually more capable of providing more continuous labor support in coordination with our nursing colleagues during the first stage of labor. The CNMs, as a whole, maintained a continuous presence when possible during the second stage and encourage resident physicians to do the same.

In our facility, nonsupine positions for second-stage labor and during birth are supported for patients who choose an unmedicated birth. These positions are also encouraged with women who have chosen epidurals as their source of pain relief. Physician trainees are discouraged from changing the patient's position from nonsupine positions to a lithotomy position for the actual birth. Most of our residents now have experience with hands/knees and side-lying births.

**Table 1**
**Number of births**

| | 2007 | | 2008 | | 2009 | | 2010 | |
|---|---|---|---|---|---|---|---|---|
| | n | % Total | n | % Total | n | % Total | n | % Total |
| **Total Births** | **2011** | | **2301** | | **2457** | | **1946** | |
| CNM-only births | 212 | 10.54 | 306 | 13.30 | 419 | 17.05 | 360 | 18.50 |
| CNM supervising intern | 130 | 6.46 | 181 | 7.87 | 282 | 11.48 | 178 | 9.15 |
| Total attended by CNM | 342 | 17.01 | 487 | 21.16 | 701 | 28.53 | 538 | 27.65 |

*Abbreviation:* CNM, certified nurse-midwife.

**Table 2**
**Type of birth**

| | 2007 (n = 2011) | | 2010 (n = 1946) | |
|---|---|---|---|---|
| **Type of Birth** | n | % Total | n | % Total |
| Primary C/S | 350 | 17.40 | 240 | 12.33 |
| Repeat C/S | 216 | 10.74 | 216 | 11.10 |
| Total C/S | 566 | 28.15 | 456 | 23.43 |
| VBAC | 25 | 1.24 | 19 | 0.98 |
| SVD | 1329 | 66.09 | 1374 | 70.61 |
| FAVD | 78 | 3.88 | 78 | 4.01 |
| VAVD | 38 | 1.89 | 38 | 1.95 |
| CNM-attended births | 212 | | 360 | |
| Primary C/S | 26 | 12.26 | 37 | 10.28 |
| Repeat C/S | | | | |
| VBAC | 2 | 0.94 | 2 | 0.56 |
| SVD | 179 | 84.43 | 321 | 89.17 |
| FAVD (referred for) | 4 | 1.89 | 1 | 0.28 |
| VAVD (either by CNM or referred for) | 3 | 1.42 | 1 | 0.28 |

*Abbreviations:* CNM, certified nurse-midwife; FAVD, forceps assisted vaginal delivery; Primary C/S, primary cesarean section; Repeat C/S, repeat cesarean section; SVD, spontaneous vaginal delivery; Total C/S, total cesarean section; VAVD, vacuum assisted vaginal delivery; VBAC, vaginal birth after cesarean.

We have also found a decrease in episiotomy rates from 2007 to 2010. In the United States, the number of episiotomies has significantly declined because of the paucity of evidence to support the routine use of this procedure without specific indications. In 2007, episiotomies were performed in 3.2% of all births. Of these, 38.5% occurred in the setting of an operative vaginal delivery. Of all episiotomies in 2007, only 3% were performed on CNM service patients. By 2010, only 1.2% of all births had an episiotomy performed; 13% of these occurred in the CNM service patients. This represents a 50% decrease in our episiotomy rate from 2007 to 2010 and correlates with a decrease in third-degree and fourth-degree lacerations (**Table 4**).

**Table 3**
**Pain management**

| **Pain Management: Practice-Wide** | n | % Total | n | % Total |
|---|---|---|---|---|
| Epidural | 1741 | 86.57 | 1244 | 63.93 |
| IV narcotics | 28 | 1.39 | 57 | 2.93 |
| No medications | 234 | 11.64 | 244 | 12.54 |
| Not reported | 8 | 0.40 | 401 | 20.61 |
| CNM-attended births (n=) | 212 | | 360 | |
| Epidural | 131 | 61.79 | 231 | 64.17 |
| IV narcotics | 7 | 3.30 | 22 | 6.11 |
| No medications | 74 | 34.91 | 104 | 28.89 |
| Not reported | 0 | | 3 | |

*Abbreviations:* CNM, certified nurse-midwife; IV, intravenous.

**Table 4**
**Perineal trauma**

| Practice-wide lacerations | n | % Total | n | % Total |
|---|---|---|---|---|
| 3rd-degree lacerations | 42 | 2.09 | 26 | 1.34 |
| 4th-degree lacerations | 6 | 0.30 | 5 | 0.26 |
| CNM-only lacerations | | | | |
| 3rd-degree lacerations | 2 | 0.94 | 1 | 0.28 |
| 4th-degree lacerations | 0 | 0.00 | 3 | 0.83 |

*Abbreviation:* CNM, certified nurse-midwife.

### *Using evidence to change practice*

In reviewing common practices with evidence to suggest a need for policy changes,[1] we have experienced a shift from continuous electronic fetal monitoring for all labor-patients to intermittent fetal monitoring or auscultation for selected low-risk patients. Because Madigan is a tertiary care medical center, labor induction for medical and obstetric indications is fairly common. In these situations, recognizing the normalcy of uncomplicated births can be difficult. Also, because we are a military facility, elective induction is often requested to allow fathers preparing to deploy or home during leave to be present for the delivery of their child. However, elective inductions are not performed before 39 weeks. Elective induction candidates must be 39 weeks, cephalic, meet ACOG dating criteria, and have a favorable cervix. Over the course of several years, collaborative practice within our facility has resulted in a greater focus of recognizing and honoring the normalcy of pregnancy and birth.

## *Collaborative Practice and Resident Education*

At the present time, we function in what has previously been described as a blended practice model.[19] As credentialed staff providers, our midwives are active and valued participants in resident education and evaluation. The ACGME allows nonphysician providers to supervise PGY-1 and PGY-2 residents when they are practicing within their scope of practice. Resident education is guided by the 6 core competencies put forth by the ACGME. The core competencies are definable, measurable methods of assessing resident progress and competency on the path to becoming an attending physician.[7]

Previous studies have noted that collaborative educational models increase collegiality and provide a sense of a shared mission.[20] One descriptive study indicated that the clinical experience and teaching ability of midwives is valued by residents and medical students.[21] In this collaborative model, continuing education is reciprocal. Physician providers provide instruction to the CNM providers in procedures that they may have less experience in performing, such as pudendal blocks, and limited ultrasounds for assessment of amniotic fluid index or first trimester dating ultrasounds. For those CNM providers interested in performing such procedures as vacuum-assisted vaginal delivery or twin deliveries, the physician staff provide education and supervision as well. Finally, CNM and physician providers often comanage high-risk obstetric patients in both the inpatient and outpatient setting. The CNM may mange the labor course of a patient with diabetes or preeclampsia, while the physician provider monitors blood sugars, and addresses glycemic control and management of hypertension.

A goal of residency education is to produce physicians who function as competent and reliable consultative providers, either to other physicians or to advanced practice nursing providers, including midwives. To that end, the core competencies of *Professionalism and Interpersonal and Communication Skills* require that residents demonstrate compassion, integrity and respect for others and that they communicate effectively with other health professionals and work effectively as a member or leader of a health care team.[22] In both our clinic and labor and delivery unit, all staff/residents/students are colocated. Thus, our outpatient and inpatient setting has a constant mix of low-risk and high-risk obstetric patients. In the spirit of teamwork, the resident, attending, and CNM providers work side by side on labor and delivery with constant cross-monitoring. When a midwifery patient develops complications that necessitate transfer to the physician team, this is generally a smooth transition.

We believe that this model of collaborative practice helps physicians in training and medical students develop respect for all levels of health care providers. By treating our CNM staff as valuable members of the faculty in both resident education and evaluation, we demonstrate the importance of their role in physician education. Further, the ability of physicians to manage uncomplicated and unmedicated obstetric patients is enhanced by exposure to the midwifery model of care. OB/GYN physicians often experience working side by side with midwives only after graduation from residency, and are therefore subject to preconceived notions of their care. By training with competent CNMs, they learn what outstanding midwifery care looks like and how to evaluate and assess the competence of care provided at all levels of care.

## Challenges to a Successful Collaborative Practice

### Lack of organizational structure

Successful collaboration requires effective teamwork and functional processes. When clear organization structure is lacking, roles blur and "gray areas" surface. Poor role clarification and failure to recognize scope of practice are 2 areas that can be overcome through on-the-spot clarification of scope of practice and clear delineation of consultation or transfer of care. Teams that have not established an adequate framework might hear comments like "I thought the midwife was just asking me a question, I didn't realize I was being consulted." When starting a new midwifery practice, early attention to the functionality of the team is important. The challenge in working with residents is that physician trainees often do not understand the scope of practice for midwives. The benefit of working in a collaborative practice environment is that residents learn to work effectively in an interdisciplinary environment, while also developing their role as a consultant.

### Poor teamwork

Effective team skills are inherent in the personalities of some individuals. However, effective teams can be developed through formal training and implementation of successful team habits requires an institutional culture shift, which must develop over time. This requires diligence and conscious adherence to the principles of effective teamwork. Otherwise, the tendency to drift back to old patterns of communication and work will occur. Key leaders must continue to promote and support the values learned in team training through risk management activities, team meetings, performance evaluation, and day-to-day communication. New employees must be formally and informally versed in the institution's team language and processes. Members who are difficult to work with can be a detriment to the success of a team. In the experience of the authors, when the culture of the organization becomes oriented toward effective teamwork, the problem member often assimilates over time. Some situations may require individual counseling, repeat training in the team model, or redress in performance appraisals. Issues of power, control and hierarchy are barriers in any team environment. Leaders can help overcome these issues by promoting team unity, and keeping focus on maintaining the horizontal relationships within the team structure.

### *Conflict resolution*

Trust and respect are maintained when disagreements are handled in a respectful and professional manner; the resolution is constructive instead of destructive. A collaborative practice does not eliminate disagreements, but they need not result in conflict. Disagreements that do progress to conflict should be resolved swiftly. Conflicts that are unaddressed, unresolved, or unjustly handled can be detrimental to the viability of a partnership and can quickly unravel the bonds of mutual trust and respect.

## SUGGESTIONS FOR THE FUTURE OF COLLABORATIVE PRACTICE

In the future, a collaborative practice model using all levels of providers (CNMs, OB/GYNs, and maternal-fetal medicine specialists) should be viewed as the ideal practice. This model should be used for both midwifery and resident education. Education in a multidisciplinary setting is invaluable for both disciplines. When considering the changes in health care that will take place in the United States in the near future, this is an opportune time for continuing study in this area. Future work could include designing models of care for the United States that use midwives as the principal primary providers of maternity care and obstetricians as specialty providers. Development of evaluation tools that assess the level of effectiveness in collaboration between care providers would be useful. We predict that successful midwife-obstetrician collaboration will be critical to successful change in the maternity care system in the United States.

## REFERENCES

1. House of Representatives Bill (HR5807). Maximizing Optimal Maternity Services in the 21st Century ("MOM'S ACT"). Women's Health Issues: 2010. Available at: http://www.whijournal.com.
2. Institutes of Medicine. Crossing the quality chasm: a new health system for the 21st century. Washington, DC: National Academy Press; 2001.
3. Milbank Memorial Fund. Evidenced based maternity care: what it is and what can be achieved. 2008: Available at: http://www.childbirthconnection.org/pdfs/evidence-based-maternity-care.pdf. Accessed January 31, 2011.
4. Carter M, Corry M, Deblanco S, et al. 2020 vision for a high-quality, high-value maternity care system. Womens Health Issues 2010;20:S7–17.
5. Institutes of Medicine. Priority areas for national action. 2007. Available at: http://www.ahrq.gov/qual/iompriorities.pdf. Accessed January 15, 2011.
6. National Defense Authorization Act, 2002, Public Law 107-107, Sec. 735, December 28, 2001.
7. Accreditation Council for Graduate Medical Education. ACGME duty hours standards now in effect for all residency programs. Available at: http://www.acgme.org/acWebsite/newsReleases/newsRel_07_01_03.pdf. Accessed January 10, 2011.
8. Baggs JG, Schmitt MH. Collaboration between nurses and physicians. J Nurs Scholarsh 1998;20:145–9.
9. American College of Nurse-Midwives. Collaborative management in midwifery practice for medical, gynecological and obstetric conditions. Available at: http://www.midwife.org/siteFiles/position/Collaborative_Mgmt_05.pdf. Accessed January 25, 2010.

10. Institutes of Medicine. Health professions education: a bridge to quality. Washington, DC: National Academy Press; 2003.
11. Nielsen PE, Goldman MD, Mann S, et al. Effects of teamwork training on adverse outcomes and process of care in labor and delivery: a randomized controlled trial. Obstet Gynecol 2007;109:48–55.
12. Nielsen PE, Mann S. Team function in obstetrics to reduce errors and improve outcomes. Obstet Gynecol Clin North Am 2008;35:81–95.
13. Agency for Healthcare Research and Quality. TeamSTEPPS®: National Implementation. Available at: http://teamstepps.ahrq.gov/. Accessed January 15, 2011.
14. Ellisngson LL. Communication, collaboration and teamwork among healthcare professionals. Comm Res Trends 2002;21(3):3–23.
15. Miller S. Midwives' and physicians' experience in collaborative practice: a qualitative Study. Womens Health Issues 1997;7(5):301–8.
16. Keleher KC. Collaborative Practice: characteristics, barriers, benefits and implications for midwifery. J Midwifery Womens Health 1998;43(1):8–11.
17. Downe S, Finlayson K, Fleming A. Creating a collaborative culture in maternity care. J Midwifery Womens Health 2010;55(3):250–4.
18. American College of Obstetricians and Gynecologists. ACOG Practice Bulletin No. 115: vaginal birth after previous cesarean delivery. Obstet Gynecol 2010; 116:450–63.
19. Collins-Fulea C. Models of organizational structure of midwifery practices located in institutions with residency programs. J Midwifery Womens Health 2009;54: 287–93.
20. Feinland J, Sankey H. The obstetrics team: midwives teaching residents and medical students on the labor and delivery unit. J Midwifery Womens Health 2008;53:376–80.
21. McConaughey E, Howard E. Midwives as educators of medical students and residents: results of a national survey. J Midwifery Womens Health 2009;54:268–74.
22. Accreditation Council for Graduate Medical Education. Common Program Requirements. Available at: http://www.acgme.org/acWebsite/navPages/nav_PDcoord.asp. Accessed January 10, 2011.

# Interprofessional Collaborative Practice in Obstetrics and Midwifery

Tekoa L. King, CNM, MPH[a,*], Russell K. Laros Jr, MD[b], Julian T. Parer, MD, PhD[b]

**KEYWORDS**

• Interdisciplinary • Interprofessional • Collaborative practice
• Multidisciplinary practice • Future of health care • Health care reform

**KEY POINTS**

- Interdisciplinary collaborative practice will be a necessary component of the health care system as it changes to accommodate more patients and become cost-efficient.
- Nurse-midwife/obstetrician teams provide seamless access for patient whose health care needs may change over the course of childbearing.
- Success of interdisciplinary teams is dependent upon professional competence, interprofessional respect, and a common orientation to the patient as the primary focus of the group.

## INTRODUCTION

Profound changes in the United States health care delivery system are anticipated as the Patient Protection and Affordable Care Act (ACA), passed in 2010, goes into effect. The ACA expands access to health care services with the goal of reducing health disparities via insurance reform, expansion of Medicaid, and mandated health insurance coverage.[1] To enact this law, the health care delivery system is faced with what may seem to be an unsolvable problem: how do we deliver quality medical services to more persons, with fewer resources? Health care services that emphasize cost-containment yet provide quality care are going to be essential in meeting the mandates of ACA.

Interprofessional collaborative practice is one model of care with a track record of providing excellent care in a cost-efficient manner.[2–4] In obstetrics, interprofessional collaboration between midwives and obstetricians also has a long history. Although midwives and obstetricians have collaborated since the inception of obstetrics as a medical specialty, only recently has the benefit of coordinated team practice been

[a] Journal of Midwifery & Women's Health, 4265 Fruitvale Ave, Oakland, CA 94602, USA; [b] Department of Obstetrics, Gynecology and Reproductive Health, University of California San Francisco, 400 Parnasus Ave, Oakland, San Francisco, CA 94143, USA
* Corresponding author.
*E-mail address:* tking@acnm.org

Obstet Gynecol Clin N Am 39 (2012) 411–422
http://dx.doi.org/10.1016/j.ogc.2012.05.009 obgyn.theclinics.com

evaluated.[5] This article reviews the literature on interprofessional collaborative practice in obstetrics, with a focus on essential components that are necessary for successful integrated practices. The term midwives refers to certified nurse-midwives and certified midwives.

## BACKGROUND

The use of interprofessional teams for the provision of health care services is an old idea that periodically comes into fashion.[2] Multidisciplinary teams often form when there is a need to provide care to persons with complex medical issues, a need to provide care to the underserved, or a need to improve a specific health outcome.[4,6,7]

### *Development and Effectiveness of Nurse-Midwifery*

Physician shortages in rural settings spurred the original development and growth of both nurse-midwives and nurse practitioners in the United States.[7,8] Frontier Nursing Service, the first nurse-midwifery practice, was implemented in rural Kentucky in the 1920s specifically to address lack of access to care with the hope of improving perinatal morbidity and mortality.[8] In 1958 the Metropolitan Life Insurance Company analyzed and published the outcomes of the tenth thousand births (selected from the first 10,000 births conducted by this service) and found a maternal mortality rate of 9.1 per 10,000, which compared with 34 per 10,000 for white women in the United States at that time. The rate of low-birth-weight infants delivered by the midwives from Frontier Nursing Service was approximately half the national average (3.8% vs 7.6%).[9]

From 1960 to 1963 a demonstration project called the Madera County Midwifery Project placed nurse-midwives in a medically underserved rural California County, hoping to improve perinatal outcomes. This nurse-midwifery practice was associated with a decrease in prematurity (11% in 1959 to 6% in 1963) and neonatal mortality rates (23.9 per 100 births in 1959 to 17.8 per 1000 births in 1963).[10] Perinatal improvements reversed when the funding stopped, and the midwives ceased practicing in this setting (prematurity in 1964–1966 was 7.4% and neonatal mortality rose to 20.6 per 1000 births).[10]

Because of the project's success, the Madera County Project was analyzed in detail and 3 key components of this project, health education, psychosocial support, and nutrition counseling, were determined to be the services most responsible for improved health outcomes. The Madera County Project then became the template for the creation of today's Comprehensive Perinatal Services Program (CPSP), an expanded service offered to women who use Medicaid funding for prenatal care in California. The core of the CPSP program is the provision of health education, psychosocial support, and nutrition counseling in addition to routine prenatal care.

### *Health Care Reform in the 1980s: Cost and Quality*

The wave of health care reform in the 1980s focused on the need to reduce health care costs, and during this time managed competition was introduced which, in short, is a form of interdisciplinary collaboration between institutions and professions.[11] The most successful of the models developed during this era of health care reform were health maintenance organizations that combined insurance and health care services. Insurance companies were also able to contract with hospitals to form preferred provider networks (PPOs), which gave the providers access to a specific pool of beneficiaries, and in exchange the insurance companies were able to lower reimbursement for individual services. The practices that thrived in this environment were those that figured out how to provide more services for less cost.

Many health care policy analysts predicted that the managed care initiatives begun in the 1980s would rapidly incorporate interprofessional collaboration among providers and expand the use of midwives and nurse practitioners. Studies that evaluated midwifery practice in terms of quality of care,[12–15] patient satisfaction,[16] and costs of care[17] all reported positive outcomes. Although midwives and nurse practitioners have become an integral accepted role within the health care team in many managed care settings, the rapid expansion and acceptance that was predicted did not materialize for 2 primary reasons, namely professional territorial battles and regulatory restrictions, which, as further explained here, still today form 2 key barriers to the expansion of collaborative practice.[18]

### *Health Care Reform Today: The Additional Goal of Patient Safety*

The current health care reform movement is not significantly different from the one that spawned managed care models 4 decades ago.[19] The goals are the same in that more care needs to be provided in a less costly manner. However, patient safety has become an additional key goal.[20,21]

The 1999 Institute of Medicine report *To Err is Human* first noted a shockingly high incidence of preventable medical errors.[22,23] In 2001 the Institute of Medicine published a subsequent analysis, *Crossing the Quality Chasm*, which evaluated deficits in the provision of health care services. This report suggested that the previous decade of health care reform efforts were an "era of Brownian motion in health care"; a not too subtle suggestion that the 1980s-1990s era of managed care demonstrated cost efficiencies but did little to improve the quality of care rendered. One of the key concluding recommendations is that all health professionals be educated about patient-centered care in interprofessional teams.[22,24]

Reviews of the root causes of obstetric medical malpractice cases consistently found that failure of interprofessional groups to work as a team and miscommunication are the 2 primary causes of preventable adverse events.[5,20,21] Evaluations of high-reliability units have also identified effective teamwork as a critical factor required for the prevention of errors.[25] In 2004, the Joint Commission recommended shared decision making and interdisciplinary teams to reduce the number of medical errors made in obstetric practice.[21]

Teamwork training via simulations of emergency events such as shoulder dystocia or postpartum hemorrhage are being implemented by hospital-based patient safety programs, but evaluation of the effectiveness of these programs is new and solid conclusions are not yet available.[26]

### *Health Care Reform Tomorrow: Add Patient-Centered Services*

The patient-centered medical home is the latest model for delivery of health care services that is expected to comprehensively encompass all the mandates of the ACA.[1] The law has a provision that funds patient-centered medical home demonstration projects, and these settings are being watched closely as they evolve. There are 5 cardinal attributes that guide the care provided via patient-centered medical homes: (1) patient-centered care, (2) comprehensive care, (3) coordinated care, (4) accessible services, and (5) quality and safety.[1] The patient-centered medical home is a team-based model of primary care, which is predicated on the assumption that a multidisciplinary team will collaborate to provide coordinated seamless care for a selected population.

Thus, over 4 decades of research on effectiveness of health care services, interprofessional collaborative practice has consistently been recognized as an important component in the provision of high-quality care. However, in the real world interprofessional practice can result in very effective collaboration and teamwork or can end in interprofessional competition and miscommunication, depending on how the practice is structured and how the individual providers within the team function.[2,6] The structure and internal processes of interprofessional collaborative practices are integral to their success.

## THE STRUCTURE OF AN INTERDISCIPLINARY COLLABORATIVE PRACTICE

Interprofessional practice has both structural and functional components of importance. Structurally, interprofessional practices can exist as midwife-physician teams in acute care settings, joint midwife-physician practices, or multidisciplinary teams caring for a specific population (ie, diabetes or adolescent clinics). In any of these settings, midwives and obstetricians can engage in parallel practices with 2 separate patient caseloads, they may share some patients with a form of consultation or collaboration, or they may function as members of a completely integrated interdisciplinary health care team with shared responsibility for one population.[2,27] In general, cost savings are more likely when the practice is highly integrated and not supporting duplication of services.

Midwives and obstetricians can act as substitutes for each other or they can provide complementary care.[13,28] When patients have direct access to a midwife for episodic or preventive health care visits, the midwife substitutes for the obstetrician and vice versa. When the midwife and obstetrician share responsibility for a single patient population, either the midwife or obstetrician will manage patients independently or both may collaborate in the management of women with specific medical or obstetric complications, depending on the needs of the practice. In this scenario, competition is avoided by careful attention to the scope of practice for each discipline and support for each other. For example, women with obstetric or medical complications will often see the midwife for health education and regular prenatal care and they will see the obstetrician for high-risk obstetric care. If the practitioners are competing for revenue, there is a disincentive to refer appropriately. However, if the providers support each other, each can offer services that result in comprehensive care for the patient without duplication or fragmentation.

For example, when the collaborative practice of perinatologists, obstetricians, and nurse-midwives formed at the University of California San Francisco (UCSF), the midwives and physicians actively looked for gaps or patient needs that were not being met. One piece of comprehensive prenatal care that was missing was patient education, as there were no standard education materials available for the patients coming to this practice. The nurse-midwives revised all patient-education materials and assembled 2 packets of education material, which are shared with the patients at the initial visit and at the 28-week visit. In addition, they rearranged their schedules so they conducted most of the initial prenatal visits, as these are the visits that are time consuming and require more orientation and education. More recently, the nurse-midwives initiated in this collaborative practice introduced group prenatal care based on the Centering Pregnancy model (Sharon Weiner, CNM, MSN, January 6, 2012, personal communication). These changes in schedule freed the obstetricians to see more women who needed gynecologic services, and freed the perinatologists to schedule more high-risk obstetric consults.

Another example can be found in the inpatient setting. Patients' discharges were being delayed for 2 reasons: they often waited for the delivering attending physician to come and sign discharge orders or they waited for an obstetrician to perform a circumcision. Because the midwives were on the Labor and Delivery unit all day, it was easier for them to do postpartum rounds for all the practice's patients and to perform circumcisions. As is often the case when a different discipline looks at a procedure, innovation occurs. The midwives learned to do anesthetic blocks when performing circumcisions, which were not at that time done at this institution. Over several years, they taught the pediatricians and ultimately, the pediatricians took over the job of performing circumcisions, all of which are now done with anesthesia.

## BENEFITS OF COLLABORATIVE PRACTICE

Interprofessional collaborative practice provides several distinct benefits for each of the players: providers, institution, and the women who receive health care services. In sharing a caseload with persons from a different professional background, individual providers gain knowledge that may not be taught within their specific discipline. For example, midwives in an integrated practice with perinatologists may learn to initially manage hypertension, autoimmune disorders, and diabetes when seeing a woman with one of these disorders at an initial prenatal visit. The midwives order initial laboratory evaluations and help the woman arrange necessary appointments in a timely manner. Conversely, the perinatologists in this integrated practice may learn techniques for delivering a baby when the mother is in a hand-knees position, or techniques used to minimize perineal tearing not taught in a traditional obstetric residency.[29] Another benefit is improved job satisfaction. In many diverse medical settings, the quality of teamwork has been positively related to job satisfaction and job retention.[30]

The institution also benefits from the interprofessional collaborative practice. Public relations and the ability to market midwifery and obstetric services without needing to fragment care can increase consumer interest in a specific institution. Interprofessional collaborative practices are well prepared to incorporate as patient-centered medical homes while institutions are remodeled to accommodate the ACA.

Meta-analyses of women's experiences with midwifery care report high degrees of patient satisfaction.[1] The most frequently cited positive experiences associated with midwifery care access to care, having a choice of provider, additional time for education and questions, and continuity of care.[31]

The benefit of lowered costs or improved revenue is difficult to delineate. Certified nurse-midwives and certified midwives have lower salaries than do board-certified obstetricians. Individual job descriptions and internal accounting decisions determine if the collaborative practice is cost-effective in any specific setting. Although it is difficult to document, an increased focus on prevention education and counseling may improve compliance with treatment requirements and lower costs via decreased length of stay and use of hospital resources.[32] Effective collaborative practice in obstetrics has been linked to improved patient outcomes, decreased length of stay, fewer cesarean sections, and lower costs.[13] Similar savings have been documented in collaborative practices in other health care settings.[26]

One more example of how the individual practice structure affects the calculated cost-effectiveness can be found in the faculty obstetrics and gynecology practice at UCSF. The nurse-midwives in this group staff the labor and delivery unit during the day. In addition to supporting the residents in the usual functions of triage, labor management, and birth, the midwives do the postpartum rounds and teach didactic courses to the medical students. Taking over these functions frees the attending obstetrician to schedule high-risk prenatal consults during the day. Postpartum rounds and didactic teaching hours do not generate direct revenue that is applied to the midwives' account, whereas prenatal consults do generate revenue assigned to the perinatologists. Therefore, this practice has an internal agreement about the value of the work done by the midwives during these hours. As interprofessional collaborative practices evolve, many different accounting models will, by necessity, evolve with them.

## ESSENTIAL COMPONENTS OF SUCCESSFUL COLLABORATIVE PRACTICE

Interprofessional collaborative practice is not comfortable for everyone. A successful interprofessional collaborative practice requires that providers in each of the relevant disciplines learn about the scope of practice of the other practitioners. Qualitative analyses of interprofessional practices have identified the following components as essential criteria for successful collaboration: (1) professional competence (common body of knowledge, shared language, similarities in treatment modalities); (2) a common orientation to the patient as the primary unit of attention, recognition, and acknowledgment of interdependence; (3) interprofessional respect for and receptivity to individual contributions; (4) a formal system of communication between providers; and (5) an effective communication based on the goal of reaching consensus (ie, an interest in solutions that maximize the contributions of all parties).[27,33–38] Detailed analyses of successful interprofessional collaboration have identified specific communication patterns and provider characteristics that support or inhibit team success.[36,39]

Team leadership deserves an important emphasis because leadership style has a substantial influence the team culture.[27] Team leaders who discourage hierarchal interactions and encourage open communication set the stage for effective communication. Very well functioning teams that have developed beyond a hierarchal structure practice a form of situational leadership whereby the clinician who is both closest to the patient and whose scope of practice is best matched to the clinical situation is recognized as the leader for that event. This role can change once or several times over a patient's overall course during pregnancy and birth. The ability of a team to function well with situational leaders is especially important in hospital-based obstetric units, which are recognized as a high-hazard industry because the work can be high-risk, high-stress, and subject to rapid changes.

## HOW CAN THEY WORK TOGETHER IF THEY DON'T LEARN TOGETHER? INTERPROFESSIONAL EDUCATION

Interprofessional education is the natural precursor to interprofessional practice, and interprofessional educational efforts have expanded rapidly in medical education over the last decade.[24,40–46] Negative stereotypes often replace mutual respect and understanding when individuals are not well versed in the cultures of their partner professions. Respect can develop best in a learning environment, yet medical students are rarely introduced to the roles of other members of the health care teams before they are required to work with these professionals.[24] Although midwifery students may have some knowledge of the obstetrician's role, a formal exposure to the professional cultures of other health care disciplines has not traditionally been a part of the curriculum in either midwifery or medical education.

Burgeoning research on acquisition of values and empathy in medical education have found that the medical school often has a "hidden curriculum" that stunts the development of empathy, secondary to a rigid hierarchal structure in combination with the preference and emphasis on biomedical knowledge and techniques.[47,48] Conversely, at least one study of the knowledge and access to evidence-based medicine by midwives based in the United States found that many had an incomplete understanding of evidence-based practice, which supports the stereotype that midwives are opposed to the use of technology or evidence-based techniques.[49]

Interprofessional collaborative education can thus serve several distinct purposes. It can familiarize individuals with the values and goals of companion professions, which can lead to improved interprofessional communication and better-coordinated teamwork.[50]

The UCSF underwent a change in the curriculum of the first-year and second-year medical students in the mid-1990s. A series of electives were developed for the first-year medical students whereby patient interaction was introduced. The nurse-midwives helped this construct and within a few years became the primary faculty for a first-year medical student elective titled A Unique Teaching Experience About Childbirth and Health (UTEACH). Medical students who chose this elective attend a series of 10 noontime lectures that address several obstetric topics such as global reproductive health, teen services, pain in labor, and the history of prenatal care. The students are paired with a pregnant woman, and attend her prenatal visits and her birth. The goal is to give the students a view of the childbirth experience from the perspective of the pregnant family and continuity of care. UTEACH gives them direct exposure to the fragmentation and contradictory advice that is often experienced by pregnant women, and helps them identify and practice ways of supporting women in labor (or anyone in pain, as the experience is eminently transferable to other acute pain settings). Two faculty nurse-midwives attend the lectures and answer any questions the students have about the care their "mom" is receiving. Several UTEACH students have matched in obstetric residencies and have continued a career in this field.

## BARRIERS AND CHALLENGES TO INTERPROFESSIONAL COLLABORATIVE PRACTICES

External challenges for practitioners in interprofessional collaborative practice are largely related to restrictions placed on midwifery practice, such as statutory limitations and credentialing requirements.[4,51] Reimbursement and internal accounting mechanisms that accurately capture both costs and revenues are the second most common challenges facing these practice models.

Certified nurse-midwives and certified midwives are licensed to practice in all 50 states, but the statutory definition of midwifery practice varies from state to state.[52–54] Statutory restrictions of importance include the degree of prescriptive authority, statutes mandating a maximum physician/midwife ratio, and statutes supporting or mandating third-party payment. However, the most important regulatory issue by far is the degree of supervision versus independent practice assigned to midwifery practice.

### *Licensed Independent Practitioners*

In some states certified nurse-midwives and certified midwives are designated as licensed independent practitioners (LIPs), whereas in others they practice under the supervision of a LIP.[51,55–57] LIP, a term coined by the Joint Commission, is defined as "Any practitioner permitted by law and by the organization to provide care and services, without direction or supervision, within the scope of the practitioner license and consistent with individually assigned clinical responsibilities." Many policies that affect day-to-day practice have their genesis in this designation.

For example, the Joint Commission allows only LIPs to have independent hospital-admitting privileges. In states where midwives practice under the supervision of an LIP, they may admit, manage, and care for a woman in labor, but there will be an added signature burden on the attending physicians for the hospital admission.

### Reimbursement for Midwifery Services

Lower reimbursement rates for midwives have historically been a significant barrier to expansion of collaborative practices in obstetrics. Until 2010, Medicare Part B paid midwives 65% of physician fee and Medicaid paid midwives at rate set by state program.[58] Thus many midwifery services have been billed under the "incident-to" provision in CPT codes, which can make accurate internal accounting difficult. Reimbursement of medical student and resident supervision has been especially complex. A full discussion of these billing challenges is beyond the scope of this article, and the reader is referred to a recent review by Wilson-Liverman and colleagues[58] for a detailed discussion of the reimbursement issues for midwives who supervise medical students and residents.

Finally, malpractice surcharges for physicians who are in clinical relationships with midwives can also provide a disincentive for collaborative practices. Malpractice surcharges are based on the supposition of vicarious liability.[59–62] In settings where the midwife is the employee of the physician, vicarious liability exists.[62,63] In settings where the midwife has an independent practice or the midwife and physicians are jointly hired by an organization, vicarious liability for the obstetrician does not exist.

In summary, the primary external challenges facing interprofessional collaborative practices are those that restrict the practice of midwifery. These barriers to practice have been slowly but consistently improving, state by state. If historical precedents can be relied on to predict the future, it may be stated with some degree of optimism that these barriers will fade more rapidly as the health care system changes in response to the requirements within the ACA.[51] It is important to remember, however, that internal barriers also exist. For example, in order to thrive, interprofessional collaborative practices require regular face-to-face meetings of group members. Dysfunction within the team may be the consequence for an organization that does not support time away from clinical activities for communication and team support.

## THE FUTURE OF INTERPROFESSIONAL COLLABORATIVE PRACTICE

The ACA may expand insurance coverage for to up to 32 million individuals who do not currently have access to primary care. Implementation of the ACA could be either a benefit or a barrier to interprofessional collaborative practice models. As managed care organizations capture a greater share of the health care market, interest in cost-effective interdisciplinary health care teams will continue to grow, but the extent to which collaborative practices are cost-effective has not been fully determined. Costs and revenue in obstetric interdisciplinary collaborative practice are difficult to delineate, given that midwifery revenue has been largely hidden in "incident-to" billing for the last decade.

Two opposing arguments address the question of how an anticipated shortage of primary care physician and nursing workforce will affect interprofessional collaborative practices, and to date there are insufficient data available to predict the outcome. First, although there is a shortage of physicians in primary care, the overall number is sufficient to meet the needs of the population. If financial incentives are changed so that more medical students go into primary care specialties and resident opportunities for primary care increase, the shortage may not materialize as expected. A glut of primary care providers may result in competition between physicians and advanced practice nurses, including midwives. However, it is not clear whether geographic redistribution, internal shifts of specialists into primary care roles, and increases in residency training programs will be sufficient to provide enough primary care physicians.

Conversely, collaborative educational initiatives currently established in several medical schools may predispose future physicians to work in collaborative practices. Similarly, staff model managed care organizations are more likely to consider increased use of nurse-midwives than are group practice organizations or private practices.

Cost-effectiveness of midwives is a double-edged sword. In most settings, the differential between salaries of midwives and physicians is significant. If physician salaries drop, the cost-effectiveness of either provider will change. Second, cost-effectiveness is predicated on effective use of midwives and physicians. The degree of delegation and the productivity of the individuals in both disciplines will affect the ultimate effectiveness of the team. How providers collaborate to maximize the skills of each will have to be assessed within the context of individual health care services. Patient acuity, overall population served, reimbursement sources, and geographic variables will affect how a practice is structured, which will in turn affect the cost-effectiveness of individual providers.

One of the arguments against the cost savings provided by midwives has been that midwives predominantly care for women at lower risk. If midwives provide care for a larger population with greater acuity, this source of cost-effectiveness may decrease. Another confounder is that the cost savings of midwives are related to a style of care that has an increased emphasis on health education and health promotion. Comparison of physician care with midwifery care is difficult because the two types of providers provide different types of care. Midwives have been found to use fewer costly resources (laboratory tests, sonograms, epidurals), and women cared for by midwives have a shorter length of stay when admitted to hospital.[15] By contrast, midwives may take longer than a physician to see a patient. Cost-effectiveness comparisons that use a direct-substitution model may inaccurately appraise the costs and/or the effects of midwifery care.

Finally, decreases in obstetric residency training programs and/or decreases in residency hours may require replacement of the current workforce. Midwives who currently practice in tertiary academic settings could rapidly fill this need.[64,65]

## SUMMARY

The 2011 revision of *The Joint Statement of Practice Relations Between Obstetrician Gynecologists and Certified Nurse-Midwives/Certified Midwives*, published by the American College of Nurse-Midwives and the American College of Obstetrician Gynecologists, affirms and recommends a high degree of collaboration between midwives and obstetricians. This relationship in clinical practice is a time-honored one, although the degree of collaboration between midwives and obstetricians can vary from minimal to highly integrated teams. Interprofessional collaborative practices that are highly integrated may be the most effective in meeting all the mandates of the current efforts in health care reform. Interprofessional collaborative practices are best poised to offer quality, patient-centered, cost-effective, and safe care.

## ACKNOWLEDGMENTS

The authors gratefully acknowledge the support of all members of the Faculty Obstetrics and Gynecology Group (FOGG) at the University of California San Francisco.

## REFERENCES


1. H.R. 3590—111th Congress: Patient Protection and Affordable Care Act 2010. February 13, 2011; HR 3590.
2. Baldwin DC Jr. Some historical notes on interdisciplinary and interprofessional education and practice in health care in the USA. 1996. J Interprof Care 1996; 21(Suppl 1):23–37.
3. Miller WL, Cohen-Katz J. Creating collaborative learning environments for transforming primary care practices now. Fam Syst Health 2010;28:334–47.
4. Institute of Medicine. The future of nursing; leading change, advancing health. Washington, DC: National Academies Press; 2010.
5. Guise JM, Segel S. Teamwork in obstetric critical care. Best Pract Res Clin Obstet Gynaecol 2008;22:937–51.
6. Fairman JA, Rowe JW, Hassmiller S, et al. Broadening the scope of nursing practice. N Engl J Med 2011;364:193–6.
7. Murphy MA. A brief history of pediatric nurse practitioners and NAPNAP 1964-1990. J Pediatr Health Care 1990;4:332–7.
8. Breckinridge M. Wide neighborhoods: a story of the Frontier Nursing Service. Lexington (KY): Univ Pr of Kentucky; 1981.
9. Joint Commission. Preventing Infant death and injury during delivery. Sentinel Event Alert Issue 30, July 21, 2004. Available at: www.jointcommission.org/assets/1/18/SEA_30.PDF. Accessed June 26, 2012.
10. Levy BS, Wilkinson FS, Marine WM. Reducing neonatal mortality rate with nurse-midwives. Am J Obstet Gynecol 1971;109:50–8.
11. Zwanziger J, Melnick GA, Bamezai A. Costs and price competition in California hospitals, 1980-1990. Health Aff (Millwood) 1994;13:118–26.
12. MacDorman MF, Singh GK. Midwifery care, social and medical risk factors, and birth outcomes in the USA. J Epidemiol Community Health 1998;52:310–7.
13. Jackson DJ, Lang JM, Swartz WH, et al. Outcomes, safety, and resource utilization in a collaborative care birth center program compared with traditional physician-based perinatal care. Am J Public Health 2003;93:999–1006.
14. Paine LL, Johnson TR, Lang JM, et al. A comparison of visits and practices of nurse-midwives and obstetrician-gynecologists in ambulatory care settings. J Midwifery Womens Health 2000;45:37–44.
15. Newhouse RP, Stanik-Hutt J, White KM. Advanced Practice nurse outcomes 1990-2008: a systematic review. Nurs Econ 2010;29:1–55.
16. Hankins GD, Shaw SB, Cruess DF, et al. Patient satisfaction with collaborative practice. Obstet Gynecol 1996;88:1011–5.
17. Cherry J, Foster JC. Comparison of hospital charges generated by certified nurse-midwives' and physicians' clients. J Nurse Midwifery 1982;27:7–11.
18. Druss BG, Marcus SC, Olfson M, et al. Trends in care by nonphysician clinicians in the United States. N Engl J Med 2003;348:130–7.
19. Bilheimer LT, Colby DC. Expanding coverage: reflections on recent efforts. Health Aff (Millwood) 2001;20:83–95.
20. Laros RK. Presidential address: medical-legal issues in obstetrics and gynecology. Am J Obstet Gynecol 2005;192:1883–9.
21. Preventing infant death and injury during delivery. Sentinel Event Alert 2004;30:1–3.
22. Institute of Medicine. Crossing the quality chasm. Washington, DC: National Academies Press; 2001.
23. Kohn LT, Corrigan J, Donaldson MS. To err is human. Washington, DC: National Academy Press; 2000.

24. de Brantes F. Bridges to excellence: a program to start closing the quality chasm in healthcare. J Healthc Qual 2003;25(2):11.
25. Mardon RE, Khanna K, Sorra J, et al. Exploring relationships between hospital patient safety culture and adverse events. J Patient Saf 2010;6:226–32.
26. O'Leary KJ, Sehgal NL, Terrell G, et al. Interdisciplinary teamwork in hospitals. A review and practical recommendations for improvement. J Hosp Med 2011. [Epub ahead of print]. http://dx.doi.org/10.1002/jhm.970.
27. Ivey SL, Brown KS, Teske Y, et al. A model for teaching about interdisciplinary practice in health care settings. J Allied Health 1988;17:189–95.
28. Stone SE. The evolving scope of nurse-midwifery practice in the United States. J Midwifery Womens Health 2000;45:522–31.
29. Ecker JL, Tan WM, Bansal RK, et al. Is there a benefit to episiotomy at operative vaginal delivery? Observations over ten years in a stable population. Am J Obstet Gynecol 1997;176:411–4.
30. Leonard M, Graham S, Bonacum D. The human factor: the critical importance of effective teamwork and communication in providing safe care. Qual Saf Health Care 2004;13(Suppl 1):i85–90.
31. Hatem M, Sandall J, Devane D, et al. Midwife-led versus other models of care for childbearing women. Cochrane Database Syst Rev 2008;(4):CD004667.
32. Butler J, Abrams B, Parker J, et al. Supportive nurse-midwife care is associated with a reduced incidence of cesarean section. Am J Obstet Gynecol 1993;168: 1407–13.
33. Brown JB, Lewis L, Ellis K, et al. Sustaining primary health care teams: what is needed? J Interprof Care 2010;24:463–5.
34. Collins-Fulea C. Models of organizational structure of midwifery practices located in institutions with residency programs. J Midwifery Womens Health 2009;54: 287–93.
35. San Martin-Rodriguez L, Beaulieu MD, D'Amour D, et al. The determinants of successful collaboration: a review of theoretical and empirical studies. J Interprof Care 2005;19(Suppl 1):132–47.
36. Sheehan D, Robertson L, Ormond T. Comparison of language used and patterns of communication in interprofessional and multidisciplinary teams. J Interprof Care 2007;21:17–30.
37. Stichler JF. Professional interdependence: the art of collaboration. Adv Pract Nurs Q 1995;1:53–61.
38. Suter E, Arndt J, Arthur N, et al. Role understanding and effective communication as core competencies for collaborative practice. J Interprof Care 2009;23:41–51.
39. Zwarenstein M, Goldman J, Reeves S. Interprofessional collaboration: effects of practice-based interventions on professional practice and healthcare outcomes. Cochrane Database Syst Rev 2009;(3):CD000072.
40. Reeves S, Zwarenstein M, Goldman J, et al. Interprofessional education: effects on professional practice and health care outcomes. Cochrane Database Syst Rev 2008;(1):CD002213.
41. Reeves S, Goldman J, Zwarenstein M. An emerging framework for understanding the nature of interprofessional interventions. J Interprof Care 2009;23:539–42.
42. Harman PJ, Summers L, King T, et al. Interdisciplinary teaching. A survey of CNM participation in medical education in the United States. J Nurse Midwifery 1998; 43:27–37.
43. McConaughey E, Howard E. Midwives as educators of medical students and residents: results of a national survey. J Midwifery Womens Health 2009;54: 268–74.

44. Cooper EM. Innovative midwifery teaching for medical students and residents. J Midwifery Womens Health 2009;54:301–5.
45. Blue AV, Zoller J, Stratton TD, et al. Interprofessional education in US medical schools. J Interprof Care 2010;24:204–6.
46. Blue AV, Mitcham M, Smith T, et al. Changing the future of health professions: embedding interprofessional education within an academic health center. Acad Med 2010;85:1290–5.
47. Chuang AW, Nuthalapaty FS, Casey PM, et al. To the point: reviews in medical education-taking control of the hidden curriculum. Am J Obstet Gynecol 2010; 203:316.e1–6.
48. Pedersen R. Empathy development in medical education—a critical review. Med Teach 2010;32:593–600.
49. Bogdan-Lovis EA, Sousa A. The contextual influence of professional culture: certified nurse-midwives' knowledge of and reliance on evidence-based practice. Soc Sci Med 2006;62:2681–93.
50. Hanson L, Tillett J, Kirby RS. Medical students' knowledge of midwifery practice after didactic and clinical exposure. J Midwifery Womens Health 2005;50:44–50.
51. Phillips SJ. 22nd Annual Legislative Update: regulatory and legislative successes for APNs. Nurse Pract 2010;35:24–47.
52. Williams DR. Credentialing certified nurse-midwives. J Nurse Midwifery 1994;39: 258–64.
53. Towers J. Status of nurse practitioner practice. Report 1. J Am Acad Nurse Pract 1999;11:343–8.
54. Osborne K. Regulation of prescriptive authority for certified nurse-midwives and certified midwives: a national overview. J Midwifery Womens Health 2011;56: 543–56.
55. Sekscenski ES, Sansom S, Bazell C, et al. State practice environments and the supply of physician assistants, nurse practitioners, and certified nurse-midwives. N Engl J Med 1994;331:1266–71.
56. Minarik PA. A vision for health professions regulation in the new millennium: recommendations from the Pew Health Professions Commission. Clin Nurse Spec 1999;13:306–9.
57. O'Neil EH. Education as part of the health care solution: strategies from the Pew Health Professions Commission. JAMA 1992;268:1146.
58. Wilson-Liverman A, Slager J, Wage D. Documentation and billing for services provided by midwives teaching obstetrics and gynecology residents and medical students. J Midwifery Womens Health 2009;54:282–6.
59. Winrow B, Winrow AR. Personal protection: vicarious liability as applied to the various business structures. J Midwifery Womens Health 2008;53:146–9.
60. King TL, Summers L. Is collaborative practice a malpractice risk? Myth versus reality. J Midwifery Womens Health 2005;50:451–2.
61. Jenkins SM. The myth of vicarious liability. Impact on barriers to nurse-midwifery practice. J Nurse Midwifery 1994;39:98–106.
62. Booth JW. An update on vicarious liability for certified nurse-midwives/certified midwives. J Midwifery Womens Health 2007;52:153–7.
63. Gilbert v. Miodovnik, 990 A.2d 983. DC Court of Appeals. 2010.
64. Angelini DJ, Stevens E, MacDonald A, et al. Obstetric triage: models and trends in resident education by midwives. J Midwifery Womens Health 2009;54:294–300.
65. Angelini DJ. Midwifery and medical education: a decade of changes. J Midwifery Womens Health 2009;54:267.

# Essential Components of Successful Collaborative Maternity Care Models

## The ACOG-ACNM Project

Melissa D. Avery, PhD, CNM[a,*], Owen Montgomery, MD[b], Emily Brandl-Salutz, MPH, MN, RN[a]

**KEYWORDS**

• Collaborative practice • Maternity care • Interprofessional education • Evidence-based care

**KEY POINTS**

- Mutual respect and trust were recurrent concepts in the collaborative practices that evolved and lasted over time; institutional culture should emphasize effective team work where all care providers are respected.
- An analysis of 12 articles describing successful collaborative practice models between obstetricians and midwives revealed common themes that can guide others planning to establish similar collaborative models.
- Regulation allowing the full scope of midwifery practice, including both state law and institutional credentialing, was essential to successful collaborative practice, although collaboration was possible in some cases where restrictive regulations remained.
- From these diverse practice settings and collaborative practice models, we provide evidence that collaborative practice not only works, but can lead to improved client and provider satisfaction and clinical outcomes.

Collaborative practice and interprofessional education are not new concepts, and have been highlighted by the Institute of Medicine (IOM) for 4 decades. These concepts and the principle of partnership were central to the recent American College of Obstetricians and Gynecologists (ACOG)/American College of Nurse-Midwives (ACNM) Joint Statement of Practice Relations Between Obstetrician-Gynecologists and Certified Nurse-Midwives/Certified Midwives[1] and the 2010 ACOG-ACNM Issue

The authors have no commercial relationships to disclose.

[a] Child and Family Health, School of Nursing, University of Minnesota, 5-160 Weaver Densford Hall, 308 Harvard Street SE, Minneapolis, MN 55455, USA; [b] Department of Obstetrics and Gynecology, Drexel University, Philadelphia, PA 19102, USA
* Corresponding author.
*E-mail address:* avery003@umn.edu

Obstet Gynecol Clin N Am 39 (2012) 423–434
http://dx.doi.org/10.1016/j.ogc.2012.05.010
0889-8545/12/$ – see front matter 

of the Year project.[2,3] The purpose of this article is to describe this ACOG-ACNM successful and sustained collaborative practices project and to report the analysis of 12 of the 60 papers submitted for the project.

The 1972 IOM report, Educating the Health Team,[4] proposed that academic health centers educate health professions students together and that other educational institutions affiliate with interdisciplinary education programs. The report further recommended that faculty become skilled in interdisciplinary teaching and model interdisciplinary practice. The IOM report authors envisioned that this cooperation would result in better use of the workforce and improvement in the quality of care.

The landmark IOM report *Crossing the Quality Chasm* provided a new focus on improving the quality of care through collaboration, recommending that our new health systems be "safe, effective, patient centered, timely, efficient, and equitable." This goal can be reached by "redesigning the way health professionals are trained to emphasize the six aims for improvement, ... placing more stress on teaching evidence-based practice and providing more opportunities for interdisciplinary training."[5(pp3,6)] Building on that work, the IOM published *Health Professions Education: Building Bridges to Quality* in 2003 and emphasized that "all health professionals should be educated to deliver patient-centered care as members of an interdisciplinary team, emphasizing evidence-based practice, quality improvement approaches, and informatics."[6(p3)]

More recently, the October 2010 IOM report *The Future of Nursing: Leading Change, Advancing Health* included these 2 important points: "nurses should practice to the full extent of their education and training" and "nurses should be full partners, with physicians and other health care professionals, in redesigning health care in the United States."[7(pp4,7)]

## ACOG-ACNM JOINT PRACTICE STATEMENTS

ACOG and ACNM have developed several statements related to joint practice over a number of years. The first was published in 1971 as the *Joint Statement on Maternity Care* and clarified that high-quality maternity care could be provided by teams of physicians, nurse-midwives, obstetric nurses, and others. The document further stated that these teams would be "directed by a qualified obstetrician-gynecologist."[8(p1)] A supplemental statement published in 1975[9] clarified that obstetrician team direction did not mean being always physically present, and clarified 3 principles:

1. A written agreement clarifying consultation and referral policies
2. Responsibility for team care accepted by the obstetrician-gynecologist
3. Arrangements for formal consultation with an obstetrician-gynecologist if team leadership is provided by a physician not trained in obstetrics and gynecology

A revised joint statement in 2001 removed the language of direction of the maternity team by an obstetrician, and referred to inclusion of an obstetrician with hospital privileges on the team to provide complete care.[10]

Recently, a more robust statement was published recognizing the common goal that obstetricians and certified nurse-midwives/certified midwives (CNM/CM) have for providing safe care to women through evidence-based care models.[1] The document clarifies that obstetricians and midwives are licensed, independent clinicians, and collaborate with each other based on client needs. It further states that care is enhanced by mutual respect and trust as well as professional responsibility.[1]

During the period of development of the 2010 joint statement, the leadership of both organizations decided to ask ACNM member midwives and ACOG Fellows with successful and sustainable collaborative practices to describe their care models in jointly written papers that could be disseminated through journal publications and presentations at the local, regional, and national level. ACOG hosted an annual competition on a clinical practice topic determined by the current president. It was through this competitive call for papers, the 2011 Issue of the Year, that the call for collaborative papers was launched by ACOG and ACNM.[2] The authors considered that highlighting the successes described by their colleagues would spur further collaboration and thus increase care options for women.

## DOCUMENTING SUCCESSFUL MODELS OF COLLABORATIVE PRACTICE IN MATERNITY CARE

A team of 3 ACOG Fellows and 3 ACNM member midwives developed the review process for the competition. Guidelines were created by this team and support staff of the two organizations. In addition to the paper having at least one obstetrician and one CNM/CM coauthor, suggested topics for inclusion were:

- Background for the initiation of the collaborative practice
- The practice model, including how patient care decisions are made
- State, regulatory, and credentialing issues that have been addressed
- Practice outcomes (using data if possible) related to women, providers, and health care setting
- Challenges faced and solutions
- Interdisciplinary education and training
- Suggestions for model replication
- Plans for any future initiatives

Clinicians from both academic and community practices were encouraged to submit papers with enough flexibility in requirements to encourage a wide range of submissions. The call for papers was issued in September 2010 through both organizations with a February 2011 due date.[3] Papers were evaluated based on thoroughness of description, sustainability, level of influence on access to care, health disparities, vulnerable populations, clinical outcomes, education, and/or research.

Sixty papers were submitted by the due date from a wide variety of practice settings across the United States. Each paper was reviewed by 2 different teams of one obstetrician and one midwife. Over a series of phone conferences, the top papers were agreed on, re-reviewed by the entire team, and finally 4 winning articles and 4 honorable-mention articles were selected. This analysis includes the 4 winning articles published in *Obstetrics and Gynecology* in September 2011[11–14] and the articles by Pecci and colleagues, Angelini and colleagues, Cammarano and colleagues, Ogburn and colleagues, Blanchard and colleagues, Egan and colleagues, Cordell and colleagues, and Nielson and colleagues describing collaborative practice models included elsewhere in this issue.

## MATERIALS AND METHODS

### *Design*

A descriptive qualitative analysis of the 12 articles was conducted to answer the question "what are successful and sustainable models of midwife and obstetrician collaborative practice in maternity care?"

### *Sample*

The sample was a subset of the 60 papers submitted: those previously published,[11–14] and an additional set selected for publication in this issue (see the articles by Pecci and colleagues, Angelini and colleagues, Cammarano and colleagues, Ogburn and colleagues, Blanchard and colleagues, Egan and colleagues, Cordell and colleagues, Nielson and colleagues elsewhere in this issue). The content analysis methodology was applied to the 4 published articles and the version submitted to ACOG-ACNM for the remaining 8 articles. An exemption from human subjects review was obtained from the University of Minnesota IRB (1201E09484). The authors of the articles agreed to have their article included in the analysis.

### *Content-Analysis Method*

A general, inductive approach to qualitative content analysis was used, as described by Thomas[15] and Hsieh and Shannon.[16] Although no predetermined codes or categories for data were used, the authors were provided with suggested guidelines to follow. These authors used similar approaches to describe their practice models, and the initial codes or categories were similar to the topics described above.

Papers were first read in their entirety to obtain a sense of the whole. NVivo 9 (software package for qualitative analysis) was used to facilitate the coding and analysis process; all articles were imported into NVivo and then reviewed line by line (M.D.A), and sections of the text were identified and coded, adding additional codes as needed. From the coded text, larger categories of related codes were derived, and finally broad themes were derived from those categories following discussion by the full research team.

Rigor was built into the process in several ways. After one author (M.D.A.) completed the initial independent coding of 4 articles, the coding was reviewed with a coauthor (E.B.S.) who had also independently coded 2 of those 4 articles. Differences in the coding scheme were reviewed and a consensus was reached. Finally, another coauthor (O.M.) independently reviewed the initial coding scheme, and differences with the original coding were discussed and consensus reached. Any possible biases or preconceived ideas in interpretation of the data were discussed in advance by the authors, and considered in discussions. Final identification of themes was discussed among all authors and a consensus was reached where differences occurred. To provide an audit trail, a record of the coding process was created, including any decisions made. As a final step, authors of 6 of the 12 articles, representing a range of practice types, were asked to review a draft of the results section of this article to determine if the summary broadly represented their experience. Overall they stated that the analysis reflected their practice model, and minor edits were made on receipt of their comments.

## RESULTS

The series of papers represented a wide range of practice locations and size. The articles are now published and may be reviewed by interested readers (see the articles by Pecci and colleagues, Angelini and colleagues, Cammarano and colleagues, Ogburn and colleagues, Blanchard and colleagues, Egan and colleagues, Cordell and colleagues, Nielson and colleagues elsewhere in this issue).[11–14] Most practices were based in urban areas and were part of larger teaching hospitals. Some practices were much smaller, including a birth center practice with a total of 5 providers. All collaborations involved obstetricians and midwives, and many included nurses and other care providers. Larger practices included advanced practice nurses and specialty physicians from areas such as neonatology, perinatology, reproductive endocrinology and infertility, maternal-fetal medicine, urogynecology, and gynecologic oncology. Academic institutions included educational collaborations with students and/or residents from the disciplines of obstetrics, midwifery, family medicine, pediatrics, and anesthesia.

Eight states were represented across the articles, namely California, Maryland, Massachusetts, New Hampshire, New York, Pennsylvania, Rhode Island, and Washington. In addition, the states of Alaska, Arizona, and New Mexico were represented as collaborative practices that are part of the Indian Health Service (IHS) and tribal health services. The number of years of practice varied widely; the oldest collaboration began in the late 1960s and the most recent in 2006.

The structures of the practices also varied. Most practices were part of large teaching hospitals, and their services were based in hospital-associated clinics and inpatient hospital units. Several practices were broader in scope; one practice comprised hospital birth services as well as 5 community clinics, a birth center, and a private practice that offered home birth. Another practice included a hospital-based office, 4 community health centers, and services at a correctional facility. In addition, 2 practices represented a combination of private practice and a federally qualified health center (FQHC) or other publicly funded clinic practice. Nearly all practices described service to women from low-income and underserved communities.

Based on the content analysis, 5 main themes were identified. Descriptions of each theme follow with quotes that amplify the descriptions provided. Some themes related to specific components of collaborative practice while others related to the formation and broader outcomes of the practices.

### *Theme 1: Impetus for New Collaboration*

Each practice described the impetus or motivation for launching their collaborative practice model. Among the reasons described were expanding practice to care for more women in a safe, cost-effective manner; providing services women were requesting such as personalized care, more female providers, and women's participation in care; offering the midwifery care model; providing learning opportunities for medical students, residents, and midwifery students; and increasing access to care for underserved populations. One alternative experience was a group of midwives who approached an obstetrician to establish a collaborative relationship. The following quotes highlight this theme.

> *Because CNMs were known to be cost-effective providers with documented success and interest in this [underserved and publically insured] population, the department initiated a 5-CNM group practice … with its own caseload of patients.*[12]

> *A large increase in prenatal registration, and a concern that the volume change would lead to an increased number of adverse perinatal outcomes, prompted the leadership of obstetrics and gynecology, its division of midwifery, and the family medicine department to address changes that could improve perinatal outcomes, patient safety, patient satisfaction, and graduate medical education (see the article by Pecci and colleagues elsewhere in this issue).*

> *This collaborative practice began … when a physician was approached by a midwife who had a successful birth center in the community [and] asked him if he would be interested in being a collaborating obstetrician. He had never met a midwife before, nor did he understand what a collaborating physician's role would entail. Recalling the advice of his residency director, strongly recommending that he work with midwives if given the opportunity, he accepted the offer (see the article by Cammarano and colleagues elsewhere in this issue).*

### *Theme 2: Basic Foundations of Collaborative Care*

Midwives and obstetricians wrote about the basic building blocks or functional components of working well together. These features included reciprocal consultation, collaborating in the care of specific clients, processes for referral of care from one clinician to another, methods of fostering clear communication, addressing any medicolegal concerns, and developing a financial structure that resulted in a lack of competition for clients and care processes or procedures. Practice guidelines were another piece of the foundation and included midwifery practice guidelines, as well as common practice guidelines used by any clinician in a given care situation. Evidence-based practice was described both as a basis for providing care and as a way of ensuring consistent management in situations where midwife clients were transferred or collaboratively managed. Regulation allowing the full scope of midwifery practice, including both state law and institutional credentialing, was described as essential to successful collaborative practice, although collaboration was possible in some cases where restrictive regulations remained.

> *Another important cornerstone to the success of the department midwifery practice was the creation of an operating agreement between the CNMs and the department physicians. This practice agreement clarifies the guiding principles and relationships between the two groups and includes the philosophy, scope of practice, functions, and organizational structure of midwifery clinical services. It details diagnostic tests and therapeutic agents that may be independently ordered by midwives, conditions requiring physician consultation, collaboration and referral, and specific protocols and guidelines.*[12]
>
> *... All members are engaged stakeholders in quality improvement activities and evidence-based policy revisions. This likely fosters consensus and group adherence to clinical guidelines, improves patient education and outcomes, promotes normal birth, and reduces medical liability.*[14]
>
> *Our collaborative practice model is possible because certified nurse-midwives in the state of Washington are independent practitioners. ... Certified nurse-midwives can admit patients under their own names, obtain full prescriptive authority, and carry their own medical liability insurance.*[11]
>
> *Decision making is shared, and is based on evidence. If a disagreement in the plan of care arises, it is discussed until the providers come to a consensus while keeping both the evidence and the woman's needs as the driving forces behind the decision. It is important to listen to the needs of the woman (see the article by Cammarano and colleagues elsewhere in this issue).*

### *Theme 3: Commitment to Successful Partnership*

The authors of the articles described additional aspects of collaboration that led to real success and strategies to solve potential problems. Mutual respect and trust were recurrent concepts describing relationships that evolved and lasted over time. Department or institutional culture should emphasize effective teamwork whereby all care providers are respected, understanding that women and their families benefit when the best of each profession is encouraged. Likewise, full participation by all clinicians in grand rounds as well as quality, credentialing, and other committees was important. Opportunities for leadership roles for both physicians and midwives were considered essential.

Faculty appointments for midwives and physicians, a seat at important tables for both, and a clear process to immediately resolve any misunderstandings are essential in supporting collaborative practice models. Midwifery and medical care models were appreciated and respected. Many practices attributed low cesarean section rates and high rates of vaginal birth after cesarean (VBAC) compared with national data, and high patient satisfaction, to their successful collaborations.

Highlights of these key aspects of partnership are evident in the following quotes.

> *...But underlying that hard work and willingness to take risks are deeper values that cannot simply be encompassed under the heading of a practice model. Shared aims, trust, and respect are the underpinnings of success at [our practice], and, we suspect, elsewhere (see the article by Cordell and colleagues elsewhere in this issue).*

> *Even among practicing obstetricians, the image and perception of midwives has been perceived as an outdated mode of practice. Common misconceptions that midwives eschew science in favor of feelings ... can be obstacles to creating an environment of trust and synergy. The reverse scenario can also be true; midwives' perception of obstetricians is that they are technology driven, are not sensitive to the needs and desires of their patients, and believe that only medically trained practitioners should provide obstetric care can interfere with the professional collaborative relationship. The truth is that midwives and obstetricians together offer the best of what maternity care has to offer. When the best of both professions are brought together in a successful collaboration, women and their families benefit.... (see the article by Nielson and colleagues elsewhere in this issue).*

> *Despite differences in the medical and midwifery models of care, the collaboration between the CNM and obstetric services ... has thrived, in large part because of a mutual respect for differences that is coupled with a dedication to common principles. Cooperation, service to the community, and collaboration in the education of the next generation of practitioners are shared core values, but respect for distinct approaches to maternity care—great minds don't think alike—has been an equally important determinant of the success of this collaboration.*[13]

> *We believe that we provide safe evidence-based care to a diverse population with varying and sometimes significant medical risk levels, and we conclude that our good outcomes are the result of our practice model and not of a high-grade, low-risk client pool.*[11]

### Theme 4: Care Integration

A shift to a common philosophy of care and committed teamwork, with the woman at the center, began to emerge in some of the practice descriptions. Care was described as each provider working to their scope of practice so that high-quality, evidence-based care was provided appropriately to women and "where the midwifery philosophy and the medical model intersect at the point of care" (see the article by Angelini and colleagues elsewhere in this issue). Care was provided to women based on their health status and care needs; separate midwifery and obstetric case loads were not necessarily required. Practice guidelines were developed and used for specific care situations rather than for specific care providers. In some higher-risk settings, midwives partnered with obstetricians in providing integrated care, resulting in improved measurable care outcomes for women. This philosophy is highlighted in the following quotes.

> *The high risk obstetrics clinic is staffed by a perinatologist, an attending physician, 2 midwives, a physician assistant and 2–3 obstetric residents. Each patient is cared for by the resident, midwife, or physician assistant, and then the case is reviewed with the perinatologist or attending physician before the patient's discharge from the clinic. The multiple providers in this model, especially the*

*stability of the midwifery and physician assistant personnel, provide a variety of benefits: to the patients, the individual providers, and our department as a whole (see the article by Egan and colleagues elsewhere in this issue).*

*When building an integrated practice, the ability of each new team member—whether physician or midwife—to work comfortably with other professionals is key. This type of practice, wherein each provider is expected to contribute to the level of their individual skills and expertise, does not work if professional hierarchies and distrust of dissimilar providers exist. This means midwives need to understand the departmental expectation that they participate in resident/student education, be willing to provide midwifery care in a high-acuity setting with relatively few opportunities for low intervention care, and understand expectations for their clinical leadership. Physicians coming in need to know midwives are not just 'present' but are actively involved in the care of women from each of the obstetric practices; the physicians must be able to build on the group expectation of mutual respect and best use of each group member (see the article by Blanchard and colleagues elsewhere in this issue).*

*This is aligned with the philosophy shared by the obstetricians, nurse-midwives, and hospital nurses who are committed to promoting spontaneous physiologic birth with the judicious use of obstetric intervention and the practice of evidence-based maternity care.*[14]

*Our collaborative model emphasizes care of the patient by a team of maternity care providers rather than a single provider. Obstetricians, family physicians, midwives and residents together review patient history, care plans and fetal tracings on every patient at formal teaching rounds in the morning and evening and informally throughout the day. This emphasis on frequent communication encourages early collaboration and discussion regarding evidence-based plans of care for each patient. All team members are encouraged to express their opinions and concerns; respectful communication is expected (see the article by Pecci and colleagues elsewhere in this issue).*

### Theme 5: Health Professions Education in an Interprofessional Practice Environment

Many of the authors practiced in settings with health professions education programs or served as clinical sites for students and/or residents, primarily obstetric residents. One article described a collaborative practice that was set up specifically to educate obstetrics and gynecology residents. Where education occurred in an interprofessional setting, residents valued midwifery teachers for their approach to normal birth and supportive teaching style; some practice sites described becoming a preferred location for student clinical experiences specifically because of the interprofessional opportunities.

*This noncompetitive, integrated educational practice model has been a successful and collaborative effort between obstetrics and midwifery using midwives as clinical faculty within an academic department of obstetrics and gynecology. The model highlights resident teaching by midwives primarily in low-risk obstetrics in collaboration with attending obstetricians in the labor unit and in the obstetric triage/emergency setting. Midwives involved in medical education are in a pivotal position to affect the education of the next generation of obstetricians and consultants while showcasing the midwifery model of care. This approach opens the door to the future of collaborative practice through innovation in obstetrics/gynecology residency education (see the article by Angelini and colleagues elsewhere in this issue).*

*Midwifery students who receive clinical training in the practice here are equally exposed to this model of care, and have the opportunity to work with medical students and residents. For example, the chief resident may review a triage plan of the midwifery student before it is presented to the faculty midwife, or an advanced midwifery student may have a medical student observe a birth and talk about why she or he makes certain choices about birth position and support techniques (see the article by Blanchard and colleagues elsewhere in this issue).*

*The birth center serves as a clinical site for those wanting to learn about the midwifery model of care including medical residents, nursing students, midwifery students, childbirth educators, and doulas. Every effort is made to offer educational opportunities and encourage a learning environment while keeping the personal, home-like environment of the birth center intact. When asked their permission first, clients are generally very gracious about allowing observation or participation of students (see the article by Cammarano and colleagues elsewhere in this issue).*

*...the interprofessional workplace and clinical training environment ...has been integral to the sustained cohesion, viability and productivity of the collaborative practice. The members of the collaborative credit interprofessional education with successes that include effective quality improvement programs, superior trainees, excellent outcomes, and longevity of the clinical service.*[13]

## DISCUSSION

This sample of the total of 60 papers submitted to the ACOG-ACNM collaborative practice project provide exciting examples of the extent to which committed clinicians are working together to provide excellent, women-centered maternity care. Although it is difficult to capture all the richness in a summary analysis, some common themes were evident. Reasons for launching the collaborative practices were provided, primarily related to a genuine desire to provide better care or increase access to care for women. Foundational aspects of collaborative practice were described. A clear description of the commitment to work together and to commit to "making it work"[12] was evident. In some cases, an emergence of a truly integrated care model with the emphasis entirely on providing the best care to women based on their needs could be documented. The number of teaching institutions in the sample provided a view of the benefits of interprofessional education settings, an idea that has been called for over the past 40 years and was the focus of a recent report led by the Macy Foundation and multiple health professions organizations.[17]

Mutual trust and respect were commonly described in these articles and have been previously identified as core to collaboration.[1,17,18] Successful collaborative care models have developed over time and have focused on client needs,[18] clinical competence, and good communication.[19] Collaboration can be synergistic and can result in quality care that has been shown to be acceptable to women.[20,21] In 1972, Meglan stated "the time has come for action,"[22(p71)] urging midwives and obstetricians to work together to improve maternity care, the same year that the IOM first called for interdisciplinary education and care.[4] The time has indeed come for more collaboration in health care among many types of clinicians. An analysis of this set of collaborative practice articles provides additional evidence that this care model can really work, describes benefits of interprofessional practice and education, and provides multiple excellent examples for others to follow.

### *Implications for Practice and Education*

The specific details in this set of articles provide a road map for those interested in developing collaborative maternity care and broader women's health practices. From these diverse practice settings and collaborative practice models, evidence is provided that collaborative practice not only works, but can lead to improved client and provider satisfaction and improved clinical outcomes. Details of the development of these practices, several in existence for more than 30 years, should enable clinicians to more rapidly develop successful practices in today's health care environment. Articulation of a clear purpose, key leaders on board to assemble the basic building blocks of the practice model, and a common philosophy with the commitment from involved health professionals to do the hard work represent an essential starting point. Policy and system-level commitments are necessary to continue to remove barriers and to address liability concerns, access to hospital privileges for all clinicians, supervisory language in state statutes, a payment model that encourages teamwork and collaborative practice, reimbursement for teaching students and residents, and a supportive workplace culture.

Numerous examples of the benefits of educating health professions students and residents together have been demonstrated in these articles. It is clear that we must work together in the education of the next generation of health professionals by partnering in assuring that students develop interprofessional practice competence in the 4 domains of: valuing interprofessional practice; understanding the complementary roles and responsibilities of one's own and other health professions; skilled interprofessional communication; and participation in team care for the benefit of the care recipient.[17]

One example of basic interprofessional education is the 1Health course at the University of Minnesota. All health professions students progress together through didactic and clinical interprofessional learning opportunities during the course of their professional programs.[23] A specific maternity care example is the Drexel University OB/GYN department transdisciplinary simulation training, hosted several times each year.[24] Midwives, nurse practitioners, obstetrics residents, undergraduate medical and nursing students, physician assistants, and anesthesia residents and nurse anesthesia students all work together on cases including shoulder dystopia, amniotic fluid embolism, and postpartum hemorrhage cases. Training occurs as an integrated team so that clinicians learn to practice together and improve the quality of care provided to women.

The concept of an integrated practice model that emerged from this analysis whereby care was provided according to women's individual needs, based on clinicians' scope of practice and most efficient use of resources, may not be a preferred practice model for all clinicians. A continuum of collaboration with an integrated model at one end of a broader spectrum of working together is described in the article by King and colleagues elsewhere in this issue. Maternity care in the United States varies by location, and a range of choices and preferences may be available: from women who may have few choices about where they obtain care, to those who may choose a specific provider and preferred care location. Some states continue to restrict the full scope of midwifery practice and, while it may be possible to work around the barrier in some settings,[13] restriction of full practice remains a barrier. Regulatory improvements continue to occur,[25] and removing these barriers should make collaborative practices more common.

### *Limitations*

This analysis represented a selection of 12 articles from the 60 papers submitted to the ACOG-ACNM collaborative practice models project. Although there were many similarities across the practices and common themes identified, it cannot be stated that these descriptions are common to all midwifery and obstetrician collaborative practices. The series of articles was overrepresented by larger teaching institutions, which may have influenced the themes identified. More information was provided about interprofessional education of obstetric residents than about other disciplines; some articles described examples of family medicine residents, obstetric residents, and midwifery students learning together. Continued analysis of the larger set of practice models may provide additional information on successful collaborative practice in maternity care. Future collaborative practices should continue to document the components that lead to success, and expand the inclusion of clinicians beyond this specific look at practices involving ACNM member midwives and ACOG Fellows.

## SUMMARY

This analysis of a series of descriptions of successful collaborative practice models provides a road map to support others in developing similar models. Midwives and obstetricians have built the necessary foundational components for successful collaborations that mature over longer periods of time. In addition, some practices provided examples of an integrated model of team care that is consistent with calls for new care models that provide high-quality care with appropriate use of health care resources.[5,17,26]

> *In the IHS, collaborative practice with CNMs and OBGs [obstetrician/gynecologists] has become the predominant model of maternity care …[providing] Native American women with high quality care that is in harmony with their culture, is cost effective, and results in improved outcomes. In a system of scarce resources, the evolution of collaborative practice has …reduce[d] adverse outcomes to low levels while achieving the positive outcomes of low cesarean delivery and high VBAC success rates …[and] is an example of how CNMs and OBGs should work together to optimize maternity care for all women (see the article by Ogburn and colleagues elsewhere in this issue).*

Obstetricians, midwives, and other health care providers have clearly moved in a direction of greater collaboration and integration in the maternity care setting. The continued development of these practices in the future is anticipated, along with increased opportunities for all health professions students to learn and practice together, with the aim of improving the health of women and their families.

## REFERENCES


1. American College of Obstetricians and Gynecologists. Joint statement of practice relations between obstetrician-gynecologists and certified nurse-midwives/certified midwives. Washington, DC: American College of Obstetricians and Gynecologists; 2011.
2. Waldman RN. Together we can do something wonderful. Obstet Gynecol 2010;115:1116–9.
3. Avery M. Call for papers on your collaborative practice models. Silver Spring (MD): Quickening 2010;41(4):27.
4. Institute of Medicine of the National Academies. Educating for the health team. Washington, DC: National Academies Press; 1972.
5. Institute of Medicine of the National Academies. Crossing the quality chasm: a new health system for the 21st century. Washington, DC: National Academies Press; 2001.
6. Institute of Medicine of the National Academies. Health professions education: a bridge to quality. Washington, DC: National Academies Press; 2003.
7. Institute of Medicine of the National Academies. The future of nursing: leading change, advancing health. Washington, DC: National Academies Press; 2010.

8. American College of Obstetricians and Gynecologists, National Association of the American College of Obstetricians and Gynecologists. Joint statement on maternity care. Washington, DC: American College of Nurse-Midwives; 1971.
9. Supplement to joint statement on maternity care. J Nurse Midwifery 1975;20:16.
10. Roberts J. Revised "joint statement" clarifies relationships between midwives and physician collaborators. J Midwifery Womens Health 2001;46:269–71.
11. Darlington A, McBroom K, Warwick S. A northwest collaborative practice model. Obstet Gynecol 2011;118:673–7.
12. DeJoy S, Burkman RT, Graves BW, et al. Making it work: successful collaborative practice. Obstet Gynecol 2011;118:683–6.
13. Hutchison MS, Ennis L, Shaw-Battista J, et al. Great minds don't think alike: collaborative maternity care at San Francisco general hospital. Obstet Gynecol 2011;118:678–82.
14. Shaw-Battista J, Fineberg A, Boehler B, et al. Obstetrician and nurse–midwife collaboration: successful public health and private practice partnership. Obstet Gynecol 2011;118:663–72.
15. Thomas D. A general inductive approach for qualitative analysis. Am J Eval 2006; 27:237–46.
16. Hsieh HF, Shannon SE. Three approaches to qualitative content analysis. Qual Health Res 2005;15:1277–88.
17. Interprofessional Education Collaborative Expert Panel. Core competencies for interprofessional collaborative practice: report of an expert panel. Washington, DC: Interprofessional Education Collaborative; 2011.
18. Keleher KC. Collaborative practice: characteristics, barriers, benefits, and implications for midwifery. J Nurse Midwifery 1998;43:8–11.
19. Miller S, King T. Collaborative practice: a resource guide for midwives. J Nurse Midwifery 1998;43:66–73.
20. Waldman R. A guest editorial: collaborative practice-balancing the future. Obstet Gynecol Surv 2001;57:1–2.
21. Hankins GD, Shaw SB, Cruess DF, et al. Patient satisfaction with collaborative practice. Obstet Gynecol 1996;88:1011–5.
22. Meglen MC. Nurse-midwives and the maternity health care team. J Midwifery Womens Health 1972;17(3):65–72.
23. University of Minnesota, Academic Health Center, Office of education. Available at: http://www.ahc.umn.edu/1health/. Accessed February 10, 2012.
24. Montgomery K, Morse C, Smith-Glasgow ME, et al. Promoting quality and safety in women's health through the use of transdisciplinary clinical simulation educational modules: methodology and a pilot trial. Gend Med 2012;9:S48–54.
25. Patrick D. MA governor's office Press Release. 2012. Available at: http://www.mass.gov/governor/pressoffice/pressreleases/2012/2012202-governor-signs-nurse-midwives-bill.html. Accessed February 4, 2012.
26. The Transforming Maternity Care Symposium Steering Committee. Blueprint for action: steps toward a high-quality, high-value maternity care system. Womens Health Issues 2010;20:S18–49.

# Collaboration in Maternity Care

## Possibilities and Challenges

Richard Waldman, MD[a,*], Holly Powell Kennedy, PhD, CNM[b], Susan Kendig, JD, MSN, WHNP-BC[c]

**KEYWORDS**

• Collaboration • Quality health care • Teamwork

**KEY POINTS**

- Collaboration among practitioners is a keystone of safe, quality maternity care, but requires thoughtful approaches to be successful.
- Collaboration is both process and outcome.
- Hierarchies and fear are major barriers to effective collaboration.
- Vicarious liability for physicians, CNMs/CMs, and NPs is a myth.

## INTRODUCTION

Collaboration can be defined in a variety of ways, including to labor together in an intellectual endeavor or to cooperate with the enemy.[1] Collaboration is a joint effort toward common goals and according to Darwin,[2] is a key factor in species survival.

Before 9/11, the United States intelligence community did not effectively collaborate with one another.[3] The Federal Bureau of Investigation, the Central Intelligence Agency, Immigration and Naturalization, the State Department, the Federal Aviation Administration, The National Security Advisor, and the White House all failed to examine security issues together, each providing their own perspective, but working collectively to safeguard the country. The result was disastrous.

The questions are whether a similar course is followed in the US maternity care and whether the highest quality and safest care is provided. Effective interprofessional collaboration is particularly important in maternity care because pregnant women move across

This article is drawn from presentations given at the 2011 ACOG Congressional Leadership Conference, the 2011 ACOG Annual Clinical Meeting, and the 2011 American College of Nurse-Midwives Annual Meeting.

[a] Department of OB-GYN, SUNY Health Science Center, 770 James Street, Syracuse, NY 13203, USA; [b] Yale University School of Nursing, 100 Church Street South, PO Box 9740, New Haven, CT 06536, USA; [c] University of Missouri College of Nursing, One University Blvd., St Louis, MO 63121, USA

* Corresponding author. American College of Obstetricians and Gynecologists, 770 James Street, Syracuse, NY 13203.

*E-mail address:* rwacog@aol.com

Obstet Gynecol Clin N Am 39 (2012) 435–444
http://dx.doi.org/10.1016/j.ogc.2012.05.011 **obgyn.theclinics.com**
0889-8545/12/$ – see front matter 

professional boundaries when they develop complications.[4] The United States is about to face a major workforce crisis in the next decade, thus interprofessional collaboration becomes even more critical.[5] The solutions are neither easy nor readily apparent. However, the crisis cannot be solved in isolation.

This article discusses the benefits and challenges of interdisciplinary collaboration in the US maternity care, reviews barriers to collaboration, and presents practical information to understand when embarking on collaborative relationships. This article also describes a recent collaborative effort between the American College of Nurse-Midwives (ACNM) and the American College of Obstetricians and Gynecologists (ACOG) in their development of a modern joint statement on practice relations.[6]

## COLLABORATION AS A PROCESS AND OUTCOME

The airline industry has identified that poor collaboration and teamwork are directly related to crashes, death, and destruction.[7] Research and subsequent actions by the industry have turned safety as a watchword and standard. They learnedto understand cultural aspects of interactions among team members and the importance of autonomy by each member to speak up in evolving situations. No one person in the team is considered infallible, and the responsibility to assure situation safety through collaboration and communication lies with each member.

Good collaboration is an additive bringing together a team that is greater than the sum of its parts through capitalization on strengths. "Individually we are a drop; together we are an ocean".[8] Collaboration is a recursive process in which 2 or more people or organizations work together to realize shared goals—by sharing knowledge, learning, and building consensus. A critical component is the identification of unifying goals through discourse and agreement together.[9]

One aspect of good collaboration is the ability to have civil disagreement. Any collaborative project should reflect the will of every one involved. Effective collaboration is maximized by open respectful honest and kind dialog. Disagreements sparked by differences can actually generate value, understanding, and in the end solutions that can be accepted by all involved as long as there are respectful and honest efforts toward resolution.

## BARRIERS TO EFFECTIVE COLLABORATION

Multiple barriers to effective collaboration are present, particularly in the complex and often very hierarchal health care settings. These barriers include a lack of understanding of interdisciplinary values, skills, and scope of practice. Inadequate knowledge about individuals in our collaborating disciplines limits the ability to effectively use available skills and talent. This inadequacy in knowledge stems from minimal cross-discipline training and rigid role expectations. The lack of collaborative ability to work in a team is common, again reflecting training and institutional hierarchal structures.[10] Day-to-day stressors and perceived insurmountable barriers of working in settings with a "this is how it has always been done" mentality can also counteract any motivation to change.

A major barrier to effective collaboration is cultural differences; all of us are socialized into roles and we have little common understanding of each other's working habits or an appreciation for each other's values. Insular cultures foster an exclusion of outsiders, which can restrict the influx of new viewpoints and reinforce one's professional beliefs. Hierarchal cultures have privilege of status, which can prevent reaching out to each other. The United States enjoys a fiercely independent and self-reliant culture, which fosters a belief that one should solve his/her own problems. Fear factors into ones actions. Many lack the confidence to ask for help; there is a fear that one will be exposed as weak. Others fear reprisal of those in power when a decision or order is questioned. Fear of litigation is a common theme across all decisions in maternity care.[3]

How can we bridge these barriers to build good collaborative teams in maternity care? How do we change culture? It requires a commitment by all and establishment of unifying goals and a common language and common value of teamwork.

These key components necessary for successful collaboration are important across and within maternity care settings. Unifying goals must be simple, concrete, incite passion, diminish competition, and establish a common fate.[3] An example in the history of the United States was President John F. Kennedy's call for landing a man on the moon after the Soviets circled the earth first. This call unified the nation and less than a decade later, Neil Armstrong took a giant step on the moon. Maternity goals can be similarly concrete, for example, setting a goal to stop all nonmedically indicated inductions before 39 weeks.[11]

## FACTORS THAT FACILITATE COLLABORATIVE PRACTICE

Specific factors that facilitate collaborative practice are professional competence, common orientation, and focus on patient-centered care, mutual respect and shared values, awareness of different roles and skills, and acknowledgment of interdependence and equality in power between individuals.[12–17] This requires recruiting the right team. Consistent communication and collaborative language, modeling, building trust, and regularly celebrating accomplishments are all useful tools in the process.

Interdisciplinary training early in careers is essential and has been well established in many academic centers, particularly in using midwives in the education of obstetric residents.[18] Interdisciplinary learning opportunities can result in a shared culture of care in the future where the woman is at the center and where there is mutual understanding of common goals. Trust and effective collaboration become the cornerstones of best care. Minimal educational strategies should: (1) prepare students for collaborative practice, (2) address health promotion and health care delivery through collaboration, and (3) promote efficient and effective woman-centered care.[19] A Cochrane meta-analysis on interdisciplinary education reported that interdisciplinary education results in improvement in the working culture, including collaborative team behavior, reduction in clinical errors, and patient satisfaction.[20] Gardner[10] outlines 10 essential lessons for collaborative partnerships (**Box 1**).

## UNDERSTANDING PRACTITIONER SCOPE OF PRACTICE

Collaborative practice in maternity care includes health professionals from various disciplines. This article discusses collaboration among physicians, certified nurse-midwives, certified midwives (CNM/CM) and nurse practitioners (NP) who provide women's maternity/women's health services.

Scope of practice refers to the health care provider's legally permissible boundaries of practice as defined by statute, regulation, and educational attainment.[21–23] The tenth amendment to the US Constitution delegates the function of professional regulation to the states, which exist to protect the health, safety, and welfare of the citizens.[22] Regulations defining the scope of practice for CNM/CM and NP vary widely by state and are the purview of different regulatory bodies.

Scope of practice laws of the state delineate the scope of practice for CNM/CMs and NPs and typically specify the amount of physician involvement required.[24] In addition to physician involvement and the authority to diagnose, prescribe, and treat, the scope of practice regulatory requirements may also include delineation of the responsibilities of the CNM/CM, NP, and physician, the presence of protocols or guidelines,

**Box 1**
**Essential competencies for collaborative partnerships**

1. "Know thyself. Each person's reality is based on self-developed perceptions. Requisite to trusting self and others is in knowing your own mental model" (biases, values, and goals).
2. Learn to value and manage diversity. Differences are essential assets for effective collaborative processes and outcomes.
3. Develop constructive skills for conflict resolution. In the collaborative paradigm, conflict is viewed as natural and as an opportunity to deepen understanding and agreement.
4. Use your power to create win-win situations. The sharing of power and the recognition of one's own power base is part of effective collaboration.
5. Master interpersonal and process skills. Clinical competence, cooperation, and flexibility are the most frequently identified important attributes.
6. Recognize that collaboration is a journey. The skill and knowledge needed for effective collaboration take time and practice. Conflict resolution, clinical excellence, appreciative inquiry, and knowledge of group process are all life-long learning skills.
7. Leverage multidisciplinary forums to increase collaboration. Being present both physically and mentally in team forums can provide an opportunity to assess how and when to offer collaborative communications for partnership building.
8. Appreciate that collaboration can occur spontaneously. Collaboration is a mutually established condition that can happen spontaneously if the right factors are in place.
9. Balance autonomy and unity in collaborative relationships. Learn from your collaborative successes and failures. Be willing to seek feedback and admit mistakes.
10. Remember that collaboration is not required for all decisions. Collaboration is not a panacea, nor is it needed in all situations.

*Data from* Gardner D. Ten lessons in collaboration. Online J Issues Nurs 2005;10(1). Available at: http://www.nursingworld.org/MainMenuCategories/ANAMarketplace/ANAPeriodicals/OJIN/TableofContents/Volume102005/No1Jan05/tpc26_116008.html.

or set specific limitations or restrictions. When entering a legal agreement related to scope of practice, all parties must be aware of the regulatory requirements for their respective disciplines within their state. **Table 1** provides examples of key regulatory issues to consider when entering into a collaborative practice arrangement.

## COLLABORATIVE PRACTICE AND MALPRACTICE RISK

Practitioners considering a collaborative practice arrangement sometimes express concern regarding liability risk. Vicarious liability refers to the liability of a supervisory party (principle) for the actionable conduct of a subordinate or associate (agent) based on the parties' relationship.[25–26] Legal imputation of vicarious liability depends on the existence of a relationship in which the principal is in control of the agent's actions and the agent is working on the principal's behalf. However, collaboration between a physician and CNM/CM or NP does not necessarily impute liability.[27] In a collaborative relationship between a physician and CNM/CM or NP, each professional functions within their legal scope of practice. The court determines vicarious liability based on the fact of each case that either support or refute required relationship elements. Proper documentation within the collaborative practice agreement can clarify the nonagent nature of the relationship between the physician and CNM/CM or NP and provide for the transition of responsibilities among independent health care providers acting within their legal scope of practice.[28]

**Table 1**
**Regulatory issues in collaborative practice**

| Regulatory Authority | Required Agreement | Provider Responsibilities | Limitations/Restrictions |
|---|---|---|---|
| • Who regulates CNM/CM/NP practice?<br>• What does the regulatory board require?<br>• How is scope of practice defined?<br>• Does the CNM/CM/NP have prescriptive authority? If so, what type?<br>• Does the CNM/CM/NP have the legal authority to prescribe legend drugs? Controlled drugs?<br>• Is special certification, education, or other documentation necessary for delegation of prescriptive authority? | • Are there requirements for a written agreement or protocols?<br>• What must be included in the writing?<br>• What should be excluded in the writing? | • What are each parties' legal responsibilities within the agreement?<br>• Must the parties practice at the same site for a designated period of time?<br>• Must the parties participate in a documentation review process?<br>• Do the regulatory entities require reports or audits?<br>• Are disclosure statements related to the type of providers in practice required to be posted?<br>• What is the delegation of backup coverage when the physician is unavailable? | • Is there a limit on the number of CNMs/CMs/NPs with whom a physician may collaborate or supervise?<br>• Is there a limit on the number of physicians with whom a CNM/CM/NP may collaborate?<br>• Are there geographic limitations on the distance between parties when care is provided? |

Although case law is most relevant to a specific jurisdiction, it can provide insight into a selected court's thinking regarding vicarious liability, as it relates to collaborative practice. This is illustrated in the *Gilbert v Miodovnik* case wherein an obstetrician provided advice when consulted by a midwife. The advice was not followed and a poor birth outcome resulted. The physician was not held liable, and the court noted that its legal conclusion was supported by public policy considerations to encourage consultation among midwives and physicians, stating, "DC has seen fit under its regulations to allow midwives to perform standard primary care for pregnant women ... encouraging the nurse-midwives to consult with obstetrics professionals is in the public interest." Imposing liability on the physician could discourage consultation.[29]

Similarly, collaboration between a physician and CNM/CM or NP does not seem to automatically lead to increased liability. ACOG surveys of professional liability from 1999 to 2003 found that the percentage of malpractice claims involving CNM-physician collaboration remained stable despite an increase in the number of physician/CNM collaborative practice arrangements.[30] NPs have lower reported licensing actions and other negative findings (occurrence rate 1 in 160 as compared with 1 in 4 for medical and osteopathic physicians). Similarly, Health care Integrity and Protection Data Bank (HIPDB) occurrence rates, which reflect fraud and abuse in health insurance and adverse payer actions, are lower for NPs (1 occurrence in 216 as compared with 1 in 21 for physicians and 1 in 19 for osteopathic physicians).[24]

## ADVANTAGES OF COLLABORATION AMONG PHYSICIANS, MIDWIVES, AND NURSE PRACTITIONERS

A recent meta-analysis of published literature between 1990 and 2008 indicates that patient outcomes following care provided collaboratively by physicians and NPs or CNMs are better in some ways than when care is provided by a single discipline.[31] In addition to improved health outcomes, a multidisciplinary approach to care is cost-effective and improves patient access to care.[31–35]

Women's health care is based on a sustained relationship between patients and their health care providers. Patients highly value the interpersonal aspects of care and may prioritize continuity of care with their personal health care provider over convenient appointment times.[36–38] However, emerging evidence suggests that current team models may not meet some patient-satisfaction measures. Studies on patient satisfaction suggest that most primary care patients experience "invisible" team care in which the roles and identities of clinicians involved in their care, such as nonphysician providers, are not clear to the patient.[37] Visible teams (teams in which the provider role is known to and understood by the patient) with a strong relationship focus are linked to higher quality primary care experiences.[39]

## THE ACOG-ACNM EXPERIENCE

The effect of collaboration on day-to-day practice must be understood. ACOG and ACNM have a long-standing history of communicating as organizations representing specific constituencies in maternity care. In 2009, in recognition of growing concerns about the maternity care workforce, the ACOG and ACNM undertook a major revision of their joint statement on practice relationships.[6] They embarked on a process that took 2 years through face-to-face meetings, teleconferences, and back room discussions to form what they considered to be unifying goals. Civil disagreement did occur, which was resolved through commitment to open honest communication and respecting each other's professional positions. For example, each organization held differing opinions about the safety of home birth, which threatened to derail efforts

**Table 2**
**ACOG and ACNM joint statement on practice relations between obstetricians and certified nurse-midwives and certified midwives (2011)**

| Statement | Rationale |
| --- | --- |
| The American College of Obstetricians and Gynecologists (ACOG) and the American College of Nurse-Midwives (ACNM) affirm our shared goal of safe women's health care in the United States through the promotion of evidence-based models provided by obstetricians-gynecologists (OB/GYNs), certified nurse-midwives (CNMs), and certified midwives (CMs). ACOG and ACNM believe health care is most effective when it occurs in a system that facilitates communication across care settings and among providers. OB/GYNs and CNMs/CMs are experts in their respective fields of practice and are educated, trained, and licensed, independent providers who may collaborate with each other based on the needs of their patients. Quality of care is enhanced by collegial relationships characterized by mutual respect and trust, as well as professional responsibility and accountability. | Safe care was a unifying concept for both organizations. We also needed to establish that we were independent providers with expertise and accountability. Finally, we agreed that quality of care was enhanced by collegial relationships with one another. |
| Recognizing the high level of responsibility that OB/GYNs and CNMs/CMs assume when providing care to women, ACOG and ACNM affirm their commitment to promote the highest standards for education, national professional certification, and recertification of their respective members and to support evidence-based practice. Accredited education and professional certification preceding licensure are essential to ensure skilled providers at all levels of care across the United States. | High standards for education and licensure were seen by both organizations as essential in standards of maternity care. |
| ACOG and ACNM recognize the importance of options and preferences of women in their health care. OB/GYNs and CNMs/CMs work in a variety of settings including private practice, community health facilities, clinics, hospitals, and accredited birth centers.[a] ACOG and ACNM hold different positions on home birth.[b] Establishing and sustaining viable practices that can provide broad services to women requires that OB/GYNs and CNM/CMs have access to affordable professional liability insurance coverage, hospital privileges, equivalent reimbursement from private payers and under government programs, and support services including, but not limited to laboratory, obstetric imaging, and anesthesia. To provide highest quality and seamless care, OB/GYNs and CNMs/CMs should have access to a system of care that fosters collaboration among licensed, independent providers. | ACNM,[b] 2011 indicates our only "civil disagreement" in that the 2 organizations have differing opinions and interpretation of the evidence on place of birth, specifically in the home. We resolved it by simply stating our positions and moving on. The statement does not commit either organization to a position in which they have to relinquish.<br>This part of the statement specifically addresses the inequities, which can preclude effective establishment of midwifery services. |

[a] A birthing center within a hospital complex or a freestanding birthing center that meets the standards of the Accreditation Association for Ambulatory Health Care, the Joint Commission, or the American Association of Birth Centers. [Foot note is from Guidelines, 6th edition].
[b] ACNM. Home birth position statement. 2011. Available at: http://www.midwife.org/ACNM/files/ACNMLibraryData/UPLOADFILENAME/000000000251/Home%20Birth%20Aug%202011.pdf. Accessed February 12, 2012.

*Data from* ACOG. Committee opinion on planned home birth. 2010. Available at: http://www.acog.org/Resources_And_Publications/Committee_Opinions/Committee_on_Obstetric_Practice/Planned_Home_Birth. Accessed February 12, 2012.

in finalizing the collaborative statement. Rather than walking away because of a non-negotiable issue, they agreed to acknowledge those differences and to step across the "line in the sand" because they believed the document was critical for future work together. It was with pride that a new joint statement approved in 2011 by both boards of directors. **Table 2** presents the statement with commentary that describes the elements of collaboration it took to reach agreement on specific points.

## SUMMARY

A shortage of practitioners to care for childbearing women in the near future is evident.[5] Collaboration may be one solution to the impending crisis.[40] Collaboration is not an accident but a well-planned and choreographed learning experience, which takes commitment, skill, cultural change, and rehearsals to bring multiple disciplines together. As in any well-constructed endeavor it takes planning, implementation, and evaluation. The major difference from the authors' perspective is that the roles become equal; all players are crucial if women, mothers, and babies are to receive the highest quality health care.[41]

## REFERENCES

1. OED. Collaboration. 2011. Available at: http://www.oed.com/view/Entry/36197?redirectedFrom=collaboration#eid. Accessed December 17, 2011.
2. Darwin C. Origin of species by means of natural selection. New York: Appleton & Company; 1877.
3. Hansen MT. Collaboration-how leaders avoid the traps, create unity and reap big rewards. Boston: Harvard Business Press; 2009.
4. Simpson KR, Knox GE. Adverse perinatal outcomes. Recognizing, understanding & preventing common accidents. AWHONN Lifelines 2003;7(3):224–35.
5. Rayburn W. The obstetrician-gynecologist workforce in the United States, facts and figures and implications. Washington, DC: ACOG; 2011.
6. ACNM, ACOG. Joint statement of practice relations between obstetrician-gynecologists and certified nurse midwives/certified midwives. College Statement of Policy. Washington, DC: ACOG; 2011. Available at: http://www.midwife.org/ACNM/files/ACNMLibraryData/UPLOADFILENAME/000000000224/ACNM.ACOG%20Joint%20Statement%203.30.11.pdf. Accessed February 12, 2012.
7. Thomas EJ, Sexton JB, Helmreich RL. Translating teamwork behaviours from aviation to healthcare: development of behavioural markers for neonatal resuscitation. Qual Health Care 2004;13(Suppl 1):i57–64.
8. Satoro R. BrainyQuote.com. Available at: http://www.brainyquote.com/quotes/quotes/r/ryunosukes167565.html. Accessed December 18, 2011.
9. Marinez-Moyano IJ. Exploring the dynamics of collaboration in interorganizational settings. In: Schuman S, editor. Creating a culture of collaboration: the international association of facilitators handbook. San Francisco (CA): Jossey-Bass; 2006. p. 869–86.
10. Gardner D. Ten lessons in collaboration. Online J Issues Nurs 2005;10(1). Available at: http://www.nursingworld.org/MainMenuCategories/ANAMarketplace/ANAPeriodicals/OJIN/TableofContents/Volume102005/No1Jan05/tpc26_116008.html. Accessed February 12, 2012.
11. ACOG. Induction of Labor. ACOG Practice Bulletin No. 107. American College of Obstetricians and Gynecologists. Obstet Gynecol 2009;114:386–97.
12. Stichler JF. Professional interdependence: the art of collaboration. Adv Pract Nurs Q 1995;1(7):53–61.

13. Miller HT, King CS. Practical theory. Am Rev Publ Admin 1998;28:43–60.
14. Miller S, King T. Collaborative practice. A resource guide for midwives. J Nurs Meas 1998;43(1):66–73.
15. D'Amour D, Sicotte C, Lévy R. L'action collective au sein d'équipes interprofessionnelles dans les services de santé. Sciences Sociales et Santé 1999;17:68–94.
16. San Martin Rodriguez L, Beaulieu MD, D'Amour D, et al. The determinants of successful collaboration: a review of theoretical and empirical studies. J Interprof Care 2005;19:132–47.
17. Suter E, Arndt J, Arthur N, et al. Role understanding and effective communication as core competencies for collaborative practice. J Interprof Care 2009;23: 41–51.
18. Angelini DJ. Midwifery and medical education: a decade of changes. J Midwifery Womens Health 2009;54(4):267.
19. Barr H, Koppel I, Reeves S, et al. Effective interprofessional education: argument, assumption and evidence. Malden (MA): Blackwell Publishing LTD; 2005.
20. Reeves S, Zwarenstein M, Goldman J, et al. Interprofessional education: effects on professional practice and health care outcomes. Cochrane Database Syst Rev 2008;(1):CD002213. http://dx.doi.org/10.1002/14651858.CD002213.pub2.
21. Bertness JA. Rhode island nurse practitioners: are they legally practicing medicine without a license. Roger Williams University Law Review 2009;14: 215–96.
22. Beck M. Improving America's health care: authorizing independent prescriptive privileges for advanced practice nurses. University of San Francisco Law Review 1994;29:951–98.
23. APRN Consensus Workgroup & National Council of State Boards of Nursing APRN Advisory Committee. Consensus model for APRN regulation: Licensure, accreditation, certification & education. 2008. Available at: https://www.ncsbn.org/7_23_08_Consensue_APRN_Final.pdf. Accessed January 8, 2012.
24. Pearson L. The pearson report. 2011. Available at: http://www.pearsonreport.com/. Accessed December 4, 2011.
25. Garner B. Black's law dictionary. 8th edition. St Paul (MN): West; 2004.
26. Jenkins SM. The myth of vicarious liability. Impact on barriers to nurse-midwifery practice. J Nurse Midwifery. 1994 Mar-Apr;39(2):98–106.
27. Winrow B. Personal protection: vicarious liability as applied to the various business structures. J Midwifery Womens Health 2008;53(2):146–9.
28. Booth JW. An update on vicarious liability for certified nurse-midwives/certified midwives. J Midwifery Womens Health 2007;52(2):153–7.
29. DC Court of Appeals. 2010. Gilbert v. Miodovnik. 990 A.2d 983.
30. ACOG. Survey of professional liability. Washington, DC: ACOG; 2003.
31. Newhouse RP, Stanik-Hutt J, White KM, et al. Advanced practice nurse outcomes 1990–2008: a systematic review. Nurs Econ 2011;29(5):230–51.
32. Chenowith DM. Nurse practitioner services: three-year impact on health care cost. J Occup Environ Med 2008;50(11):1293–8.
33. Thompson M, Nussbaum R. Asking women to see nurses or unfamiliar physicians as part of primary care redesign. Am J Manag Care 2000;6(2):187–99.
34. Office of Technology Assessment (OTA). The cost and effectiveness of nurse practitioners. Washington, DC: U.S. Government Printing Office; 1981.
35. Lenz EM. Primary care outcomes in patients treated by nurse practitioners or physicians: two year follow-up. Med Care Res Rev 2004;61(3):211–4.
36. Safran DG, Murray A, Chang H, et al. Linking doctor-patient relationship quality to outcomes. J Gen Intern Med 2000;15(Suppl):116.

37. Safran DG, Wilson IB, Rogers WH. Primary care quality in the Medicare Program: comparing the performance of Medicare health maintenance organizations and traditional fee-for-service Medicare. Arch Intern Med 2002;162(7):757–65.
38. Safran DG. Defining the future of primary care: what we can learn from patients. Ann Intern Med 2003;138(3):248–55.
39. Rodriquez HS. Attributing sources of variation in patients' experiences of ambulatory care. Med Care 2009;47(8):835–41.
40. Waldman R, Kennedy HP. Collaborative practice between obstetricians and midwives. Obstet Gynecol 2011;118(3):503–4.
41. Collins-Fulea C. Models of organizational structure of midwifery practices located in institutions with residency programs. J Midwifery Womens Health 2009;54(4):287–93.

# Index

*Note:* Page numbers of article titles are in **boldface** type.




Obstet Gynecol Clin N Am 39 (2012) 445–451
http://dx.doi.org/10.1016/S0889-8545(12)00068-X

**N**

Printed and bound by CPI Group (UK) Ltd, Croydon, CR0 4YY
03/10/2024
01040460-0009